9 UNTOLD SECRETS TO PAIN-FREE BREASTFEEDING

GET A DEEPER BOND WITH YOUR BABY WHILE COMBATTING ENGORGEMENT, SORE NIPPLES, TONGUE TIE, AND LOW SUPPLY

KIMBERLY NICOLE WHITTAKER

CONTENTS

I dedicate this book to my children and all mothers who stood for the great cause of breastfeeding. Breastfeeding is a great fight, but I would like to uplift those mothers who didn't give up, steadfast, and prevailed. Salute to all strong mothers; you are loved and appreciated!

INTRODUCTION

Motherhood is a wonderful journey. The emotions that come with it are unexplainable, from that joyous moment when you become aware that you are carrying a bundle of joy inside you to the point when you finally get to stare into your baby's beautiful eyes after nine months of anticipation. At that point, all you just want to do is to give your baby the best things in the world. If only it were that easy! The harsh reality is that even when we have the best intentions, caring for our newborns can be challenging.

Medically, exclusive breastfeeding, especially during the first six months of birth, is recommended as the ideal and natural way to supply our babies with all the required nutrients they need to grow well and boost their immune systems. Of course, none of us want to deprive our babies of such benefits intentionally. However, breastfeeding is a journey with ups and downs. But why should mothers experience this in the first place?

Well, the truth is that most of us are just ill-informed about the different challenges that come with breastfeeding. So, it is

Just going to a movie theatre to watch *Titanic* without your crying tissues with you. Okay, this is a lovely way to put it, but you get the idea. There is so much we need to understand about breastfeeding, but the thought rarely crosses our minds.

Many people believe that being strongly motivated is essential for successful breastfeeding. That is very true! Nevertheless, lactation problems occur even among women with the highest motivation to succeed at breastfeeding. So, what does that tell us? It's simple and straightforward that breastfeeding is psychological and physical when it comes to proper execution. Now you might be thinking, "How exactly does that work?"

I'm glad you asked! That question is precisely why I am writing this book! The contents will expose our minds to essential details about the breasts and their anatomy. By understanding the breast and its anatomy, we will better understand the processes involved in milk production. Don't worry. It won't be another biology class. Now, once we internalize adequate knowledge about the anatomy of the breast and the formation of lactation, it becomes effortless for us to learn how to breastfeed and better nourish our babies from the start properly. It seems like magic, isn't it? Maybe!

This book also covers common breastfeeding questions and addresses concerns that most new moms tend to have, especially during the early days of breastfeeding. Together, you and I will walk through a week-by-week and stage-by-stage overview of breast milk development. This is to help you become very familiar with the outsides and the insides of your breasts.

It doesn't end there! We will also look at practical information on common lactation challenges and strategies to overcome them. More than that, the book approaches all these breastfeeding issues from a body-conscious perspective.

As mothers and women, understanding the anatomy of the breast and the other areas mentioned above lays a better foundation for proper breastfeeding. It also guides us to understand the true powers of our bodies. This is something many of us don't even realize exists. With this knowledge, we will understand the problems we face, where they originate from, how to fix them, and explain them to those who can help us solve them.

I know this seems like a lot, but we will take these steps together, hand in hand. I got you.

When I carried my kid for nine months, I wanted the very best for my baby, not once thinking I would have issues breastfeeding. So, I had no option but to learn on the job - the hard way. It wasn't easy. I have had only one easy breastfeeding journey, but then I had a breast reduction which caused all of my struggles with my last two children. These experiences made me realize how important it was for women and new moms to become aware of the challenges involved in breastfeeding quickly early. All the information I will share with you will help you and every new mama out there, to prepare and become capable of overcoming any challenge in the best way. Most importantly, I hope to help you so that your complications won't negatively affect your mental and physical health. Your mental health is another critical priority on our list of objectives.

I think that is that point where I'm supposed to take a pause to properly introduce myself. So, I am 'Kim.' I was born in Kingston, Jamaica, though I now live in the sunny state of Florida with my husband and three lovely children. I have a newborn baby girl, a five-year-old girl, and an eight-year-old boy. A fun fact about my family – we are all fully vegan! I breastfeed all of my three children! Seasoned mamas here would agree that is a whole lot of experience!

Like every other breastfeeding story, you might have heard before, it was quite challenging, especially with the last two – my baby girls. Of course, there had to be a reason. I had breast reduction surgery! Wait for what? Yes! You read it right! I decided to get a breast reduction as I was very large at that time. During the procedure, my areolas were completely removed. Little did I know that this would alter my ability to produce milk and properly breastfeed my babies. Now, I bet you must be thinking, "Wow! So, what happened next?" Well, you would have to come along with me on this adventure to see how things turned out for my babies and me. You don't have to worry, though; it has a happy ending.

Now hear me out: I want you to know that it's not something you should feel guilty about when it comes to breastfeeding issues. Do you think it is your fault? No! Rather, it is the minimal guidance that prevents you and other women out there from achieving good milk production and a euphoric breastfeeding experience. So, it's not your fault. Sometimes, our bodies just work differently.

To the moms-to-be about to start this journey with us, I need you to know that you have already earned the title of the World's Best Moms. It doesn't matter if you haven't officially become one. Seriously, I am not exaggerating here.

Do you know why? By picking up this book to read, it shows that you've decided to become intentional about your growth. Believe me, that action alone has helped set up the first foundational layer you need to succeed in your breastfeeding journey.

Just a little disclaimer! Everyone experiences a unique breastfeeding journey. So, if your neighbor goes through a specific breastfeeding challenge, that doesn't mean you will experience the same. This common misconception is why we will ensure that you gather as much knowledge so that you will understand yourself better. However, you must know that your determination to make your experience better is as important as the ideas provided in this book. We need both to make this work!

Every woman deserves to enjoy the pain-free experience of being a new mom with brighter smiles and healthier looks. It will be a long ride. Ensure you are comfy, with your mind settled, and ready to reflect! Grab popcorn or something. Are we done? Great! Now, let's get this journey started!

GETTING TO KNOW YOUR BREAST

*Y*ou might be thinking, "So, what else could I possibly not know about my breasts? Come on; I have been dealing with them since puberty hit me, right?" Well, I can assure you that you wouldn't be asking the same thing at the end of this chapter. You must know what the anatomy of your breasts precisely constitutes, as well as the creation of breast milk. This is not necessarily a secret. However, a good understanding of your breast will help you make the most of the 9 secrets I will share with you. So, it is chapter 1 – our best chance to make the most solid foundation for a remarkable breastfeeding journey! Let's get started!

ANATOMY OF THE BREAST

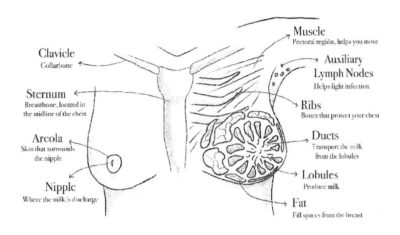

Before we even proceed with this, let's do a breakdown of the phrase, 'anatomy of the breast'; it means the different structures within our breasts. So, let's do a quick pre-test; how many parts of your breast can you identify correctly? Of course, I can't hear your responses, but keep them in mind and grade yourselves as we continue.

The female breast is a paired structure of specialized tissues overlying your pectoral muscles, which simply means your chest. These specialized tissues have three major classifications; fatty tissue, connective or fibrous tissue, and glandular tissue. The fatty tissue is the amount of fat in your breasts; it determines the size of your breast. The fatty tissues are also called adipose tissue, and they form a large portion of our breasts. Like you might have already guessed from the name itself, the connective tissue and ligaments perform the function of connecting the skin of your breast to the pectoral muscles. It also provides support to the breast and gives it its shape. It kind of balances the fatty tissue. Now to our primary focus for the whole of this book - the glandular tissue! This body component is also known as milk-producing tissue. Now so that you know, these three classes of tissues don't just exist on their own. We can find them in different breast structures, which leads us to ask the next and most important question, "what makes up the anatomy of the breast?"

The first thing we need to get familiar with is the breast mammary glands. These glands make mammals (organisms that breastfeed their offspring) 'mammals.' Does that make sense? The production of the mammary glands is a result of the modification of our sweat glands. They begin to develop early in embryologic life and only culminate during postpartum lactation. So simply put, you are born with them, and they continue growing till your breastfeeding stage. Another essential feature you need to know about the mammary glands is that the endocrine system regulates them. They become functional in response to hormonal changes. Whew! So many scientific details, right? Let's switch things up.

Usually, the mammary glands may signify the primary symbol of femininity. Guess why? Their active presence in our breasts is what makes us different from males. So basically, they are non-functional in male breasts but functional in ours. Apart from that, the mammary glands are the fundamental structures involved in lactation. So here is how it works; since we said earlier that the glandular tissue is the milk-producing tissue, the mammary glands are milk-producing glands that house the glandular tissue.

Now about the glandular tissue! From now on, please note that each of your breasts contains 15 to 20 lobes of glandular tissue. All of the 20 lobes radiate around your nipples like spokes on a wheel. I'm going to need your rapt attention here because things are about to get a little complicated. But not to worry, I've got you! So each lobe is subdivided into many smaller structures, called lobules. The lobule is precisely the main site for producing breast milk. The lobules contain alveoli, which are tiny grape-like sacs made of milk-secreting cells. Now we know the structures responsible for producing milk, so how does it get to be suckled by your baby?

Nestled amidst the other components of the glandular tissue, we have the milk ducts. These ducts are responsible for transporting the milk. Now the movement doesn't just happen like that. The breast contains a basket of smooth muscle cells called myoepithelial cells surrounding the alveoli – the milk-making sacs. When the myoepithelial cells contract, they squeeze the milk out of the milk-making glands and through the tiny tubes of the milk ducts. So basically, the milk ducts are tiny tubes that transport the breast milk from its point of production in the alveoli to the nipple openings. Your baby directly sucks to draw out milk. So we can think of the milk ducts as individual straws, sometimes merged, which end at your nipple to transport milk to your baby. We have about eight to nine of those straws.

Finally, we have the visible parts of the breast that most of us probably only know about – the nipple and the areola. Let's start with the nipples. They are located right at the center of your breasts. Each of our nipples is composed mainly of smooth muscle fibers. If you've been following well, you would not be surprised to hear now that each of your nipples has about 15 to 20 openings for milk to flow. The female nipple has a rich network of nerves. I bet some of you will agree with that because sometimes we get so frustrated at how sensitive our nipples and breasts are as a whole, even at the slightest touch. Blame those nerves, sisters! Apart from making your nipples sensitive, these nerves also send signals to the brain to stimulate the release of breast milk and more milk production. You will get to see exactly how that works when we discuss lactation physiology.

Next, we have the areola. Don't raise your eyebrows at the

name just yet! You see that circular disk of roughened pigmented skin that surrounds your nipple, right? That's what is called the areola. There are also numerous small bumps on the areolae surface, which are called Montgomery's glands. These glands secrete an oily substance that acts as a protective lubricant for the nipple. They darken and enlarge during pregnancy which means more oil to moisturize the nipples and areola.

The breast also contains lymph vessels, blood vessels, and lymph nodes. As the name implies, the blood vessels circulate blood throughout the breasts, chest, and body. This blood usually contains oxygen and other nutrients that are important to the cells in the breast. On the other hand, the lymph vessels transport lymph, a fluid that helps your body's immune system fight infection.

And that is it for the anatomy of the breast! Now that we have analyzed the different components that make up the breast more internally and externally, let's see how they function in milk creation. But a quick check to be sure we are both on the right path. In this chapter, we discussed the functions of the major components of the mammary gland, glandular tissue, as well as your nipples and the nerves within them. If you have understood all of this, then we are good to go!

THE LACTATION PHYSIOLOGY

A common misconception that most of us tend to have is that the size or shape of our breasts determines our ability to produce milk or breastfeed. This assumption is not true at all! While your breast size can be an inherited trait or result of surgery or other factors, breastfeeding success has nothing to do with it. So let's throw that thought in the trash as soon as possible.

Now, did you know that your breasts have been preparing

for your pregnancy and breastfeeding journey right since you were in your mother's womb? Not possible, right? Well, it is! When you were born, your mammary glands and ducts, which transport milk out of your breasts – had already formed. These glands stayed dormant until you hit puberty. That is when the magic happens!

Some particular hormones regulate the mammary gland's function. At puberty, our estrogen and progesterone levels begin to increase. Each of these two hormones has specific functions. Progesterone induces duct system development. The increasing estrogen levels promote the growth of the mammary glands and glandular tissue in your breast. You may not believe this, but increased estrogen also causes your breast to increase in size by accumulating adipose tissue. Guess we now know how puberty does the magic of growing your breast, right? You will also notice an increase in the size and tenderness of your breasts each month after ovulation. That is to show you how your body and breast prepare for pregnancy and breastfeeding. If there is no pregnancy, the fullness and tenderness subside, and the cycle repeats.

However, when you become pregnant, you are bound to notice so many changes in your breasts. The progesterone and estrogen hormones cause the milk ducts and milk-making tissue to increase in shape and size. These pregnancy hormones also cause the breast to change in composition. The developing mammary glands from puberty shift into high gear; they further develop. This reaction is just to show that estrogen and progesterone are indirectly involved in lactation.

After giving birth, the pituitary glands release two hormones that directly affect breastfeeding - prolactin and oxytocin. The pituitary gland secretes the hormone prolactin using its anterior lobe. However, its posterior lobe does the job of secreting the hormone oxytocin. The prolactin hormone from the anterior pituitary stimulates milk production within the glandular tissue, and oxytocin causes milk ejection from the glands. Too much to take in, isn't it? Let's break it down!

Prolactin causes your alveoli to take nutrients such as proteins and sugars from your blood supply and turn them into breast milk. So we can say that prolactin is the hormone that directs the alveolar sacs. While discussing the anatomy of the breast, we talked about how the myoepithelial cells contract around the alveoli to eject your breast milk through the tubes of the milk ducts. Of course, the cells cannot just acquire on their own and without help. Oxytocin is the hormone responsible for promoting that milk ejection and the let-down reflex.

Funnily enough, the production of oxytocin can also be triggered by something. Tiny nerves are activated in the nipple when your baby suckles your breast. Remember, we talked about how your nipple is a powerhouse of nerves. These nerves send sensory impulses from the nipple to the brain, cause the oxytocin hormones to release into your bloodstream, and the final result is pushing out or letting down the milk. Oxytocin also causes the muscles of your uterus to contract during and after birth. With this specific function, it helps your womb to get back to its original size. Oxytocin can even help reduce bleeding after childbirth. An important point here is that both prolactin and oxytocin are hormones that can help you as a mother to form an emotional bond with your baby.

All of these that we just discussed make up the different stages of lactation physiology. The normal physiology of lactation is a process that begins to take effect well before the initial latch of your newborn baby. As you have read, these stages of development, from puberty, pregnancy to lactation itself, are influenced by a collection of physiological changes. Nonetheless, each of these developmental stages is essential for successful breastfeeding.

If you wonder whether there is possibly anything that can distort this normal physiology of lactation, the answer is "yes."

Such an occurrence could be responsible for a mother's body not making an adequate amount of milk for her baby, even when everything else is in order. This particular condition is called primary lactation failure. It can be due to different factors, including previous thoracic or breast surgery, which may affect critical nerves or ductwork. It could also be a result of hormonal complications such as polycystic ovarian syndrome or thyroid abnormalities. These are conditions in which the mammary tissue simply did not develop during adolescence. We will get to understand more about this in the next chapter!

But first, we all deserve to applaud ourselves because guess what? We have completed our first foundational layer. So, let's proceed with the building process.

MILK PRODUCTION AND HOW TO INCREASE IT

*A*s soon as your baby is born and the placenta is delivered, the brain releases the hormones prolactin and oxytocin. Do we remember what prolactin and oxytocin hormones do? The magic of breast milk – production and ejection, isn't it?! Once the prolactin signals your alveoli to make plenty of milk for your new baby, the oxytocin then directs the muscles around the alveoli to squeeze milk out through the milk ducts. Now, many processes fall in between those two hormonal actions we just described. However, you need to know that your breasts begin to produce milk between 16-22 weeks of your pregnancy.

This chapter will spice things up slightly by analyzing the milk production process, focusing on the frequently asked questions that most mamas tend to ask about milk production. Sounds exciting, right? Let's get started!

WHEN WILL I START PRODUCING BREAST MILK?

One of the greatest surprises I encountered after giving birth to my first daughter was the incredible amount of time it took for my breast milk to come in. Now using the phrase, "come in," I mean the time it took for me to notice a significant increase in the volume of my breast milk and changes in its composition. Keep this phrase in mind because you will see more of it. Now back to my story, I was more confused than surprised. Even though I had read beforehand that it will take an average of two to five days for that to happen, I couldn't help but wonder, "So how am I to feed and offer my baby the nutrients she needs with just tiny drops of this fluid? Come on! It isn't white in color!" I know the experienced mamas reading this right now will be like, "Oh, I know that feeling." In the end, I learned that it was normal.

As moms, we shouldn't expect to get large milk volumes in the first few days after birth. Remember we mentioned earlier that milk starts from about the 16-22 weeks of pregnancy? The milk your breast produces at that time is the colostrum! Colostrum is the early concentrated pre-milk that the breast offers. Many medical practitioners termed it - liquid gold. Why? Because it is so low in volume yet so dense in nutrients and disease-fighting antibodies. The colostrum also stimulates your baby's first bowel movement and reduces the risk of digestive upset. No exaggeration intended, but colostrum has everything your newborn needs in the early days after birth until your later milk becomes present.

Now how are we even sure that the liquid gold will be sufficient for your baby? Well, at the time of birth, your baby's stomach is tiny - most likely the size of a walnut. As such, your baby probably won't need more than a few teaspoons of this 'liquid gold' per feeding. Besides, in the first few days, newborns tend to sleep a lot to survive solely on the colostrum.

Because the colostrum may not be leaking or easy to express, many mothers may not know that their breast is producing this early milk. However, for some mamas, things are entirely different. The colostrum begins to leak right from the last weeks of their pregnancy. Another point of difference is that the colostrum may be thick and yellowish for some women. In contrast, it may be thin and watery for others. Whichever category you fall into, you are good to go!

WHEN CAN I EXPECT MY BREAST MILK TO INCREASE?

Biochemically, the transition from colostrum to mature milk is usually between 30 and 40 hours after delivering the placenta. I know what you're thinking, "but I didn't experience that!" Yes! That's because it will take a little while for the changes to become apparent to you as a mum.

Unlike what most of us mamas think, colostrum doesn't just transition into mature milk. In between the colostrum and mature milk production, we have transitional milk, which is usually the color of the regular milk mixed with orange juice. When do you get to see this change? It is usually about 3 or 4 days postpartum. Though studies have shown that transitional milk tastes a lot better to your baby, it contains less immunoglobulin and protein than colostrums. Nonetheless, transitional milk makes up for that reduction by providing your baby with more lactose, fat, and calories instead.

The next and final stage of milk production is the arrival of mature milk! All things being equal, this milk starts to arrive about 6 -12 days after postpartum. So what's its composition? Your mature milk is usually whiter in color, though it can be slightly bluish sometimes. Also, it is more like watery skim milk. Like you would expect, the mature milk packs a more signifi- cant amount of fat and other nutrients that your babies need to grow. Perhaps, this explains why you will begin to see an increase in your baby's weight when your mature milk starts arriving.

So how exactly would you know that you are in high gear

KIMBERLY NICOLE WHITTAKER

within 30 - 40 hours after you deliver the placenta? Has breast milk increased? Honestly, that is something that you cannot miss. You will see why I said so in a bit.

The first thing you may notice is that your breasts will start to feel full and heavy. This fullness and heaviness is called breast engorgement. It comes with a bit of tingling and dull ache. Now you can see why I said it's something you cannot miss. Want to know something even more enjoyable? Some mamas do not feel any of these sensations, which doesn't mean something is wrong with them. I kind of wish I was one of them, though. I'm just kidding! Anyways, the initial heaviness and pain will ease once your body adjusts to a regular breastfeeding and pumping routine.

The veins in your breasts will become more pronounced, and your breast milk may drip and leak more. This time, you will notice that the milk that leaks is no longer thicker and golden colostrum. Instead, it will be thinner and whiter. Your nipples may also become flattened, with the skin around your areolas becoming tightened and firm.

The signs of gradual change are not only restricted to your breast. You may also notice a difference in your baby's feeding patterns and behavior at the breast, especially in the amount of milk they consume.

WHAT IF MY BREAST MILK DOESN'T COME IN EARLY?

I cannot overemphasize that every mama's timing is different, be it pregnancy or milk production. However, I made it clear earlier that your body's breast milk production begins to work fully within thirty hours after you deliver the placenta. Some studies have proven that the timing of your milk increasing in volume is completely controlled hormonally.

Now, how do we translate that into plain English? Your

mature milk coming in depends on hormonal changes taking place in your body during that moment. If your breast milk takes longer to go in, you don't have to worry. I'm not trying to patronize you. Even world-renowned scientists and medical doctors have confirmed that many mothers experience their milk coming in as a gradual change rather than sudden and very noticeable. Research shows that about 35% of mothers may take longer than five days before their milk begins to come in.

If you still can't help but worry, here is an explanation to make things more straightforward for you. When your breast milk does not increase in volume as expected within three to five days of birth, that situation is termed "Delayed Onset of Lactation or DOL." Several factors may be responsible for this condition.

It could be because you had an exhausting labor experience, notwithstanding the mode of delivery. It could be a prolonged pushing stage during vaginal birth or an emergency cesarean section. Intense blood loss during labor may also pose a problem.

Mamas who have gestational diabetes or any other diabetes that require treatment with insulin may also experience DOL. The reason for this is that any fluctuation of blood sugar after you've given birth can have an impact on how fast and efficiently your breasts make milk. There is a way out, though! It would help if you tried to breastfeed as often as you can. Doing this will help stabilize your blood sugar which makes it easier for your breasts to produce milk.

Retained placenta or anything that affects placental function can also cause DOL. Though having retained placenta is quite rare, you should make sure to seek the help of your midwife as soon as possible if you experience any symptoms of the retained placenta, such as continued heavy bleeding and tummy cramps after your delivery. All you need is a minor procedure to remove the placenta fragments. And voila! You're fine! Breast surgery or injury that involves either the damage or removal of specific breast tissue may also interfere with the milk production and ejection process.

Above all, you need to understand that even with all the factors we just mentioned, your milk is most likely to come in when it's time and on schedule! So, you don't have to be scared of anything!

WHAT CAN I DO TO INCREASE MY BREAST MILK?

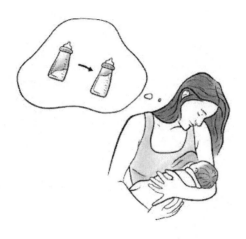

ESSENTIALLY, what we are about to discuss is not limited to mamas dealing with Delayed Onset of Lactation but every mama in general. At the initial stage of my first breastfeeding journey, the nurses in the hospital advised me to feed my baby every two hours, even when I objected that I didn't think she was getting anything. According to them, the more she suckled, the faster colostrum would transition into mature milk. What these nurses were trying to teach me was that breastfeeding was a supply and demand process.

So, in essence, our babies play very significant roles in our milk production process. Here is how it works. Your baby suckles and removes milk from your breast, right? Good! So each time your baby feeds and empties your breast milk, the prolactin hormone gets the signal from the nerves on your nipple and then directs the body to make more milk for the next feeding. The logic here is that the more milk your baby demands to drink, the more milk your body will produce and supply. One of the best ways to encourage your baby to drink more is through skin-to-skin cuddles, which involve you snuggling with your baby.

If you still haven't gotten the idea, what we mean is that the amount of milk your breast produces will vary according to how much your baby eats. By breastfeeding for as often and as long as your baby wants, you are indirectly helping your body to make more milk. Initially, you might feel like you are doing nothing but breastfeeding. But eventually, you and your baby will transit into a breastfeeding pattern that works for both of you.

Apart from the fact that frequent breastfeeding, especially in the first few days and weeks of your newborn's life, can help you increase your milk supply, here are a few other ways that you can consider for a good milk supply;

For a start, you can try hand-expressing milk to your baby. What does that even mean?! Well, it simply involves you using your fingers to collect drops of colostrum from your nipple and then feeding your baby. To make it easier, you should start by massaging your breasts and then move on to finger-feed your baby with the drops of milk from your breasts. Some mamas even use a syringe to collect the milk.

A warm compress can be of great help too! All you have to

do is to place it on your breasts before you start nursing your baby.

You can also schedule an appointment with your doctor or certified lactation consultant to give medical advice on how to increase your milk production and monitor the baby's health progress.

As much as possible, you should try to be relaxed. You can consider going to a calm and gentle place to help you with that. Always remember that you can't feed and care for your baby properly if you are not in a relaxed and comfortable state.

WHAT SHOULD I EAT DURING PREGNANCY AND AFTER BIRTH TO PRODUCE MORE MILK FOR MY BABY?

Using a scale of 1 to 10, how often have you heard someone talk to you about how her milk supply shot up after she started eating something for breakfast, lunch, or even desserts? I'm sure it's at least probably an eight, maybe nine if you're a first-time mom. Of course, it cannot be charming sometimes. But you can't blame them because some specific foods and herbs have been proven to an extent to be very helpful in promoting a more excellent milk supply. Though there is only limited scientific evidence to back these claims, some of the experienced mamas here, including myself, can testify that these foods encourage more breast milk production. By the way, galactagogues are the medical term for describing food sources and drugs that help increase our breast milk supply. Galactagogues shouldn't be too hard to pronounce, right? Well, let's examine five galactagogues scientifically verified to be safe and effective for breastfeeding mums.

. . .

1. Fenugreek Seeds: Unless you live under a rock, you would have heard about fenugreek. It is a quite popular option when it comes to increasing breast milk production. Or perhaps you may have seen them without knowing! Several studies, including a 2018 study conducted with 122 breastfeeding mothers, revealed that these aromatic seeds have great potentials of significantly increasing the amount of milk produced by nursing mothers. Now you might be wondering, "What exactly makes these tiny seeds so powerful?" According to these researchers, the fenugreek seeds contain estrogen-like compounds, which are great for enhancing milk flow. So how much of these fenugreek seeds can you take to get effective results while keeping yourself and your baby safe from side effects? You can start by steeping half or one teaspoon of whole fenugreek seeds into a cup of boiling water and then allowing it to sit for about 15 minutes before sipping at least two or three times a day. If you haven't figured it out yet, we just explained how you could make fenugreek tea! You can also explore your culinary creativity by finding ways to include these seeds in your vegetables or meat dishes. Or you can blend them with other fruits to make smoothies. Some mamas even go for a more concentrated form of fenugreek, which is the capsule supplement. A little warning, though; some moms who use fenugreek have reported that though it increases their milk supply, the seed seems to make their babies gassier.

2. Oatmeal or oat milk: Ever heard of desserts called lactation cookies? Indeed, you can draw out their usefulness from the name, right? Well, there are high possibilities that these milk-boosting cookies contain a good amount of oats. Apart from that, oats, be it in the form of the traditional oatmeal or a trendy oat milk latte, have been a go-to option for breastfeeding moms to make more milk. I can even confirm the benefits of these nutritious gems. Though there is not much scientific evidence to prove its actual effects, oats have an impressive nutrition profile. Wouldn't you be amazed if I told you that only half a cup of dry oats offers around 20 percent of the iron content that breastfeeding moms need per day? Isn't that a lot? So, if you haven't tried it out, you should!

3. Garlic: Quick question; are you by any chance allergic to garlic? If your answer is a yes, then step to the side and give us a minute! Now for the mamas that can tolerate garlic in their diet, you should know that eating it in moderation is not only beneficial but can stimulate and increase your milk supply. However, you must note that the garlic you eat, whether raw or in your foods, travels into your milk. Thus, its solid and pungent odor can alter the smell and taste of your breast milk. Now, this isn't just about you; your baby must be comfortable with its aroma and taste. If your newborn is not bothered by any of this, then feel free and enjoy using a moderate amount of garlic to flavor your dishes be it vegetables, meat, pasta, or seafood

4. Lean meat and poultry: Like I stated earlier, iron is an essential mineral that can help promote an increased milk supply for your baby. So as the latest mama in the city, you can include top sources of iron like lean beef, pork, lamb, and poultry into your diet, and thank me later! Just make sure that it isn't undercooked before eating.

5. Fennel seeds: My last breast milk supply booster is a very traditional galactagogue that has been in use for centuries! If you haven't tasted them before, let me give you an idea! Fennel seeds are crunchy seeds laced with a unique licorice flavor.

They are very similar to the fenugreek seeds in several ways. First, the former contains the infamous estrogen-like compounds, which help in enhancing milk supply. A handful of small studies have also shown that fennel seeds are associated with increased milk volume and fat content. Just like the fenugreek seeds, you can make fennel tea or use its seeds as a flavoring agent in your salads, sauces, vegetables, and even soups. Oh! They are also available in capsules!

"In all things, practice moderation!" This statement should be our watchword as you try out some of these galactagogues! The early stage of your delivery can easily be the most frustrating part of the newborn days for you. Still, with the overly long list of tips that you and I have deeply discussed in this chapter, we can slowly begin to transform our breastfeeding experience for the better.

HOW TO BREASTFEED

*S*o far, you might be wondering why we had to go through two entire chapters before finally discussing this much-anticipated topic 'How to breastfeed'. Well, learning the basics about the breast and its milk production system in chapter one and chapter two will make it easier for us as we explore and uncover some of the secrets to having the most fantastic breastfeeding experience, whether you're a first-time mama or an experienced mama.

Apart from your pregnancy, your breastfeeding stage is another stage where you get so curious and unsure of the actions to take concerning your baby. Questions like - "How many times a day do I feed my baby? Is there a breastfeeding schedule or technique that you should follow? What if he/she is sleeping? Should I ever wake my sleeping baby to breastfeed?" – constantly pop up in your mind. Dear mamas, let's take a deep breath in and relax because, in this chapter, we will provide answers to all of these common questions while at the same time giving our first-time moms the best idea of what it looks, sounds, and feels like to breastfeed.

WHEN IS THE BEST TIME TO START BREASTFEEDING MY BABY?

Ideally, it is better to start nursing within the first few hours of your baby's birth. The reason for this is that babies tend to be extremely alert in those first few hours of their lives. Thus, by breastfeeding right away, you can take advantage of this natural wakefulness. When you miss that opportunity, then it might be harder to get your baby to breastfeed adequately. Why? You would notice that newborns usually take their time sleeping for most of the next 24 hours. Though they look so cute while sleeping, feeding them at that point is almost impossible!

HOW CAN I TELL IF MY BABY'S HUNGRY AND READY TO FEED?

Interestingly, somebody had asked me this question before I became a mother. My instant response was, "Oh! That's simply when my baby starts crying". Unfortunately, that mentality of mine did not change even when I got blessed with my first pregnancy. Like I said in my introduction, I had to learn even this on the job – the hard way. Of course, I'm not alone on this, but now we know better!

Dear mamas, you must understand that crying is a late sign of hunger. It is most likely that point where your baby has gotten uncomfortably hungry and upset. Two problems can arise when this happens. First, it cannot be easy to calm your little one down. Also, newborns tend to use a lot of energy when they cry, and this will surely make them tired.

If any or all of the problems happen, then your baby might not breastfeed as well as they should. They might fall asleep before they finish feeding. Of course, we don't want any of these happening. So, let's not wait for the tears: our babies might be tiny and unable to speak, but there are many ways they can make their needs known, such as:

- Sucking furiously on their hands, fists, or even on your shirt and arm as you hold them.
- Moving their head from side to side
- Opening their mouth or puckering their lips as if to suck
- Sucking on their lower lip or tongue - when they do this action, it can look like they are sticking their tongues out
- Making all kinds of lip-smacking sounds
- Nuzzling against your breasts
- Have you ever heard of the rooting reflex? It's that moment when babies open their mouths and turn their heads, usually in the direction of something that's stroking or touching their cheeks which they assume to be food.
- Even if your baby does cry as an early sign of hunger, it will probably be just a short, low-pitched wail that rises and falls.

Just like their mamas, every baby is different. So, your baby may show some or all of the hunger cues mentioned above. It is alright if you don't know precisely what your baby's hunger cues are at first. But as the days go on, you will begin to recognize and get familiar with your baby's specific hunger cues.

HOW DO I LATCH BABY ONTO MY BREAST?

Having learned how to detect when your baby is hungry, the next paramount question is 'how do you satisfy that hunger?" It's time for another one of my stories. So, after giving birth to my first child, doing all the necessary documentation and check-ups, we went home happy. I had no idea until about three days later that my baby wasn't latching correctly. He was sucking on the end of my nipples. This action wasn't allowing him to get enough milk, and at the same time, it made me sore. Like many new moms here, I thought or perhaps assumed that babies often come inherently wired with adequate knowledge on how to latch on and breastfeed correctly. What a myth! Some weeks later, I came to understand that a proper latch is not easy to achieve. It was a period of trials and errors for me. Oh, I forgot to add a time of having sore nipples!

But wait! I can feel some first-time mamas already raising their eyebrows at me with a question: what do you mean by "latching on"? So, let's take it from the top. Latching on means the way your baby takes your nipple and areola into her mouth to suckle. Always keep in mind that the emphasis is on both the nipple and the areola. Latching is the most important aspect of breastfeeding.

So why is it so essential to master the act of good latching? It is simply the core foundation of your successful breastfeeding experience. First of all, it saves your nipples from soreness which is very important. It also enables your baby to feed freely and stop once he/she is satisfied. Also, a good latch translates into your breasts getting stimulated to produce more milk. But what happens on the other end of the tunnel? Improper or inadequate breastfeeding latch opens doors of frustration and distress for both you and your baby. Not only will you have to deal with sore nipples as I did, but your baby may suffer poor weight gain due to the inability to drain your breast effectively. A poor nursing latch may also reduce your milk supply, thereby putting you at increased risk of blocked milk ducts and mastitis.

You don't have to be scared, though, because we will be unveiling some simple steps that should help you get on track in your latch-on skill so that your babies can get all the nourishment and comfort they need. But first, you must check your baby's latch with a breastfeeding expert before leaving the hospital. I wish I did that much earlier; it would have saved me a lot of trouble. Now that we have gotten that out of the way let's see what this step-by-step guide is about!

1. Start by holding your baby right with the front of her body facing yours, tummy to tummy. Her mouth should also be meeting your breast with her head in line with the rest of her body. This setup will help make swallowing easier.

2. Once your baby is well-positioned, hold your breast with your free hand and tickle her lip with your nipple. This action will encourage her to open very wide. If she still doesn't open up, try squeezing some milk onto her lips. In case she turns away, gently stroke the closest cheek- side to you. By doing that, you can activate the rooting reflex, which will make her turn her head toward your breast.

3. Once her mouth is wide open, bring your baby forward, ensure your breast and aim your nipple just above her top lip. Make sure you resist the temptation to lean over and push your breast into her mouth. Instead, allow your baby to take the initiative and find your nipple.

4. Keep hold of your breast until your baby latches on firmly and begins to suckle well. Make sure that your baby's mouth covers both your nipple and the areola. That way, her mouth, tongue, and lips will easily massage milk out of your milk glands. Sometimes, you might see that a part of your areola is not inside your baby's mouth. That's fine because the size of our areola and baby's mouths differ. But here is a little tip that works; you can gently shape your breast as you bring your baby to feed!

9 UNTOLD SECRETS TO PAIN-FREE BREASTFEEDING

5. Good job so far, but it's not game over yet! Now watch out and listen to ensure that she is not just sucking on her own lower lip or tongue or gumming your nipple. There are different ways you can use to know this. Firstly, you can try pulling her lower lip down while nursing. Then observe to see if she is exhibiting a robust and steady suck-swallow-breath pattern. At first, she might start with a short and fast suck to stimulate your milk flow, but once you feel your milk coming in, listen to the sound of her swallowing or gulping the milk slowly and deeply with pauses in-between. However, if all you hear are clicking noises, you should know that something is wrong with your baby's latching position. If your baby is indeed suckling well, you will also notice a rhythmic motion in her cheek, jaw, and ear. But if all of that is in place, then we are good to go.
6. Remember to support her neck, shoulders, and hips as she suckles.
7. If your baby still latches on the tip of your nipple or the latching hurts, just gently insert a clean finger in your little one's mouth to break the suction. Then start the lip tickling afresh, gently letting your baby latch on again correctly, with both the nipple and the areola in her mouth.

Here are other signs you should watch for to be sure whether your baby is doing a correct latching position.

- Firstly, the latch should be as comfortable and pain-free as possible.
- Your baby's chin and the tip of her nose should be touching your breast. She should also be comfortable breathing through her nose.

- Her lips will be flanged out, like that of a fish, rather than being tucked in.

Anytime you are having trouble getting your baby to latch correctly, try observing your environment. If it is too noisy, try moving to a quiet, calm place where your baby can fully concentrate on feeding. Also, remember the kind of magic that skin-to-skin cuddles can do to your baby's appetite. Just make sure that in every breastfeeding session, your baby takes the lead!

To our lovely mamas with inverted nipples, though I don't want to scare you, I must let you know that adequately latching your babies is a bit more difficult for you. But keep in mind that the word is difficult, not impossible! Of course, anything that is difficult can be made easy! You can make use of a nipple shield or shell between feedings to make it easier for your baby to suck from your nipple. Pumping is a beneficial method too. If you are not sure how exactly to go about it, not to worry, we've got you covered with a whole chapter that you and I will be exploring very soon.

HOW LONG DO I BREASTFEED?

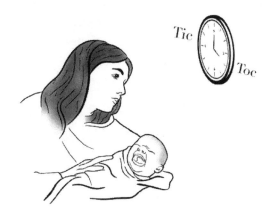

I don't know about the experienced mamas here. Still, before my first baby and even till now, I have heard people say that feeding babies for long can cause soreness and crack in our nipples. Honestly, that is false. Soreness or nipple cracks are conditions that arise when you employ an improper or a less-than-ideal latching position when breastfeeding your baby – a reminder that we all should take the lessons from the previous section very seriously.

Now back to the feeding length, it is ideal to allow your newborn to breastfeed for as long as he/she will stay on the breast, especially in the first few days and weeks of birth. So instead of setting time boundaries on each feeding session, allow your little ones to take their time at the breast. The only thing you have to do is check out for the signs that your child is satisfied. These signs are undoubtedly the only ways to ensure that your baby is getting enough breast milk at each feeding session.

Besides, breastfeeding your baby longer is also a plus for you as the mama. Remember, I said in the previous chapter that the more often and the longer you breastfeed your newborn, the larger your breast milk supply. So, while ensuring that your baby is well-fed, you also get to stimulate your milk production and build up your breast milk supply! How is that? Here are some additional tips that can help you determine how long to breastfeed your baby;

EXERCISE FLEXIBILITY: On average, breastfeeding sessions last between 20 and 30 minutes. But keep in mind that every baby is different; thus, they could spend more or less time feeding. In the initial stage and during the growth spurts, it might take longer for your baby to feed. So, you can try feeding your newborn for about 10 to 15 minutes on each breast. This time is likely to reduce as your baby gets older because he will drain the breast faster.

FOCUS ON DRAINING **one breast fully:** If you are one of those mamas who believes that your baby must feed on both breasts by all means during every feeding session, then we must talk! You see, contrary to popular belief, it is more important and ideal that at least one of your breasts is well-drained at each feeding. The last drops of the mature milk, which we refer to as hindmilk, are richer in fats and calories. Hence your baby stands to gain more if allowed to feed on the hindmilk. So, wait till your baby drains one breast before offering the other. If he falls asleep or doesn't want to anymore, then don't force it! Start breastfeeding your baby with the other breast during your next nursing session.

· · ·

ALWAYS WATCH **out for the baby to confirm her satisfaction:** If there is anything we have learned from the latching process, then it is the fact that your baby calls the orders here. You can only end the feeding when she is ready to. Typically, you would expect your baby to let go of the nipple when she is satisfied, right? Well, because she is a boss baby, she might decide not to. It is now your job to find ways of figuring out whether your baby is satisfied or not. To make the job easier for you, here are a few cues that can help you confirm when your baby is happy and ready to end the feeding session.

- He stops breastfeeding on his own and turns away from the breast.
- His suck-swallow patterns will slow down to maybe one or two sucks per swallow.
- Your baby falls asleep, and your breasts feel emptier.
- He appears content.

Whichever means you use to confirm that your baby is satiated, ensure that you break the latch gently. There are two techniques with which you can do this; press on your breast near the baby's mouth gently, or you should try inserting a clean finger into the corner of your newborn's mouth and break the suction.

HOW OFTEN DO I BREASTFEED?

If you had the option of picking between feeding your baby on-demand or on a schedule, which would you like? Many of us would most likely go for the latter because it is more convenient. However, the best option to ensure our breastfeeding success is to nurse our babies on demand, that is, when they're hungry. Beyond that, staying flexible with your baby's feeding schedule helps to ensure that you feed her whenever she shows signs of hunger. It also provides your newborn with a sense of comfort and security.

Since your baby is born with a small stomach and a lesser appetite, there are high chances that they won't demand much feeding. Nevertheless, you should feed your baby at least 8 to 12 times a day, every 24 hours. If we break that down, you will probably be breastfeeding your baby every two to three hours, day and night.

We would want to make this pattern the general feeding timetable for every baby, we can't. The reason for this is that feeding patterns vary in an extensive range from baby to baby. You might find yourself nursing a little more or less frequently. Take, for instance, my baby might be the hungrier and more impatient kind. At the same time, yours is a more easily satisfied infant. We both definitely can't employ the same time interval in feeding our babies, right? While I may go for just a little more than an hour between feedings, you might be able to enjoy three-and-a-half to four hours in between each feeding session. It's all ball down to the uniqueness of each baby.

Now I know I said earlier that the small size of your baby's stomach might lower his/her demand level, especially in the first few days and weeks. Having a smaller stomach also means that breast milk gets easily digested. That should explain why your baby may want to feed many times in a short period. Nonetheless, your baby's feeding pattern may start to change when she begins to grow, and your milk supply increases. Since her stomach gets bigger and she consumes more milk, your baby's body takes longer to digest the milk, which will, in turn, allow her to take extended breaks between feedings.

One thing you should understand is that breast milk can be more easily digested than infant formula. You can't compare your baby with that of your neighbor who consumes formula or other solid supplements. The formula-feeding baby will eat far less often than your own breastfed baby, whose tummy gets empty faster.

There is no better way to end this chapter than to remind you that breastfeeding is one of the most challenging and yet most fruitful things we do as new mums. I know that all of these things we have discussed so far are easier said than done, but you know what? You are not an ordinary mother but a super mama. So, whatever you do, do not let it drag you down. By investing the right amount of patience and practice, you will quickly become a breastfeeding expert.

DEEP LATCHING AND POSITIONING

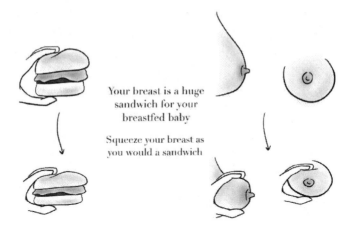

Your breast is a huge sandwich for your breastfed baby

Squeeze your breast as you would a sandwich

bout a month ago, my girls and I were having a hangout. Somehow, the discussion about our breast-feeding experience popped up! As we were recounting our adventures and teasing each other, one of my friends just said,

"You know guys, before we all became mamas, we assumed that getting our breasts to produce lots of milk for our babies was the most important part of breastfeeding! I wish I had the chance to go back in time; I would have also focused well on observing and learning the best ways to position and latch my baby on." And we were all like snapping fingers because you know what? She said it all!

In the previous chapter, you and I went through a little step-by-step latching process that is quite effective for your baby. Consider that a trailer! In this chapter, we will be unveiling the full movie! Deep latching! Remember, we explained that latching refers to how your baby takes your nipple and areola into her mouth to suckle. Now find a way of making the word "deep" reflect that definition. Let me help you with that – deep latching involves doing a latch appropriately while ensuring that your baby gets the maximum milk intake at every feeding. So basically, the opposite of this is the shallow latch where your baby isn't getting enough milk, yet you feel pains and discomfort.

Before we even explore the world of deep latching, you must understand that certain things have to be in place before you even can achieve this kind of latch. That foundational element is your positioning! What is that? It simply means how you hold your baby as you attempt to breastfeed her. Proper positioning is necessary to encourage and get your newborn to latch on the very moment you offer her your breast. Also, it helps eliminate chances of any breastfeeding problem, especially nipple soreness. So, you want to get a proper deep latch that looks good, feels comfortable, and delivers effective results, right? Let's get you stuffed up with the necessary information about all the breastfeeding positions that can work best to get you and your baby ready for deep latching.

BREASTFEEDING POSITIONS

As usual, I have something to add before we get into the discussion about the different breastfeeding positions. It's an introduction that is long overdue! If you're ready, permit me to introduce you to every nursing woman's Brest friend real quick. Yes! The spelling is B-R-E-S-T!

As a new mom, a proper pillow is the kind of Brest friend you need, especially in the first few days of your breastfeeding journey. You can gain a lot of benefits with the sort of added structure and support that it offers. Now you might be wondering, "what if I get so used to the pillow? How will I learn how to nurse without it?" You will learn just fine as time goes on. But for the first few weeks of breastfeeding, you need a pillow to show kindness to your neck and your back. All of these breastfeeding positions can be more comfortable when you use your Brest Friend! Now let's see how you should do these breastfeeding positions!

CRADLE HOLD: As a new mom, you will most likely be taught the essential cradle hold right from the hospital. Perhaps, that explains why most of us experienced moms are particularly very familiar with the breastfeeding position. If you have no idea of the way we do the cradle hold, stick with me, and let's go through it step by step. And if you're an experienced mama like me, it wouldn't hurt to relearn.

- Start by sitting upright while holding your baby. Her head should rest in the bend of your elbow of the arm on the side you will be breastfeeding. So, if you are breastfeeding your baby on your right breast, her head should be resting in the bend of the left elbow.

That same hand should be supporting the rest of her body.

- Next, cup your breast with the other free hand and then compress it gently with your thumb above your nipple and areola. You should place your index finger at the spot where your baby's chin touches your breast. If you are doing it correctly, then your nipple will point slightly toward the baby's nose. And your baby is ready to latch and feast on a deeper level.

Though the fact remains that the cradle hold is one of the most common breastfeeding positions, that doesn't mean that it is perfect for you and your baby. So, let's see what other breast-feeding positions can work better for you and your baby.

CROSS CRADLE HOLD: This position is just like the cradle hold, but your arms should be in a different position this time. This particular position can give you adequate control over how your baby takes the breast into his or her mouth. With this control, you can get your baby to latch on more deeply! To do the cross-cradle hold;

- Start by holding your baby's head with the hand opposite to the breast from which you'll be nursing. For example, if you are nursing from the right breast, you will support your baby's head with your left hand.
- Place your wrist between your baby's shoulder blades and lift his mouth towards your nipple with your thumb behind one ear, your third finger very close to the other ear. You may also need to use a pillow on your lap to raise your baby to a nipple level.
- Now cup your breast as you would for the cradle hold, using your free hand. And get ready to latch.

Football hold: This football hold, which is also the clutch hold, is especially helpful for those mamas among us who went through a c- section and would not want to place their babies against their abdomen as they breastfeed. It can help if your baby was born premature or if you have a beautiful set of twins. But wait, why am I even recommending this particular position for you? Well, see for yourselves!

- To breastfeed your baby in a football hold position, start positioning him at your side with him facing you.
- Then tuck the newborn's legs under your arm on the same side as the breast from which you're nursing. Are you now getting to know the origin of the name football?
- Once that position is well set up, support your baby's head with the same hand, and finally, use your other hand to cup your breast and point your nipple to your baby's nose, as we learned with the cradle hold.

Now you see that you would not have to touch your abdomen through the breastfeeding session.

SIDE-LYING POSITION: For our first-time mamas who may not know this, permit me to inform you that there is no way you wouldn't have to breastfeed your baby in the middle of the night. As such, this same breastfeeding position can be an excellent choice. Now how is it done?

- Lie on your side with your pillow beneath your head. Also, lay your baby on his side so that he will be facing you. Your baby's head should be in line with your nipple and his tummy to your own.

- You may want to use your hand from the other side to cup your breast. Doing this might make it easy for your baby to latch correctly.
- You may also place a small pillow behind your baby's back to protect her and hold her close.

Before we proceed to the last one, you must understand that this position works well when you are on a bed. That's why it is a good choice for nighttime. So, under no circumstance should you try it on a couch, recliner, or even a water bed! Another thing to note is that excess beddings shouldn't surround your baby because they can cause her to suffocate. So only one pillow is enough to hold her close. Adding anything more can pose a problem.

LAID-BACK POSITION ("BIOLOGICAL NURTURING"): If you want a breastfeeding position suitable for both your couch and your bed, then this is it! With this position, you breastfeed your child while leaning back comfortably on a semi-recliner or a sofa. You can also apply it when you are in bed, but most likely with pillows to support your upper back, neck, and head. Just like the cradle hold, the laid-back position is also an excellent breast-feeding position for your newborns. It is a highly recommended nursing position for mamas who have smaller breasts. Also, suppose your little one is excessively gassy or has a super-sensitive tummy. In that case, you might want to consider trying out the lad-back position! Here is how it works.

- First, you should lean back on a bed or couch, with your body well supported by pillows in a semi-reclined position.
- Place the baby on you, tummy to tummy. Your baby

should be resting on your chest. Make sure your baby is lying in a comfortable direction. The only thing you should be concerned about is for the whole front of your baby's body to be against yours. Your reclining body should also support his weight.

- Interestingly, this nursing position takes advantage of gravity and naturally allows the baby to seek your nipple and latch on. Notwithstanding, you can also help your newborn by holding your breast and directing the nipple toward his mouth for more accessible and deeper latching.

- Once your baby is well-positioned and ready to latch on your nipple, all you have to do is to lie back and relax. You can even use your free hands to caress and cuddle with your little one. Nothing feels good like a mama's touch.

OF ALL THE breastfeeding positions discussed in this chapter, there is no 'right' or 'wrong'! What do I mean? A practical and comfortable deep latch is what we seek, right? Well, only you can tell if a particular breastfeeding position is offering you those two benefits. You will know that a latch is effective if the baby produces an adequate number of dirty diapers in a day. Suppose he is gaining weight after a few days. In that case, he demands breast milk about 8 to 12 times a day, and most importantly, he seems satisfied after every breastfeeding session. So dear mamas, no matter how overwhelmed you are with information, always remember that you are the best judge of what is helpful. If it doesn't feel comfortable and painless to you, then it isn't the best! So, ignore the excesses and be confident in using what feels suitable for you and your baby!

HOW TO DO A DEEP LATCH WHEN BREASTFEEDING

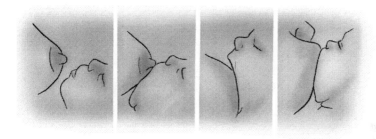

Since we have already learned the different breast positions that can help you set up the foundation for a deep latch, let's find out the best ways you can do a deep latch. So, let's assume that you are already holding your baby, whether in a cradle, crossover, laid-back, side-lying, or football position, and then we will take it from there.

- Hold your breast and place your index finger and thumb on the edge of the nipple. Squeeze the two fingers together and get your breast compressed. Your other fingers should be kept off to the sides so that it's like you are pinching just an inch.
- Now gently bring your baby's mouth to the breast by supporting his head with one hand, your thumb on one side of the ear, and your third finger near the other ear. At the same time, the web of your hand should be supporting the nape of your baby's neck.

Slightly tilt his head by using the heel of your hand to lift between his shoulder blades.

- Now that your baby's head is tilted back and his chin facing uplift him to touch your nipple. The nipple should be resting just above his upper lip. Remember, your baby runs the show here, so wait until he opens his mouth wide and then places your breast first into his lower jaw.

- Next, tip your newborn's head forward and place his upper jaw behind your nipple. As you place the upper jaw behind your nipple, ensure that you press your thumb down to form the 'flattened sandwich.' By doing that, you can make your baby's lower jaw more deeply positioned than the upper jaw.

- Now your work is done! Just wait for a few seconds and then release your breast from your fingers. Sometimes, you will notice that your baby's nose deeply presses against your nipple; tilt his head slightly so that you can see his nose because it is still in contact with your breast. Once that is done, you don't have to press your breast with your fingers anymore.

NOW WE UNDERSTAND that the process of delivering milk from our breasts to the belly of our babies demands a great deal of knowledge and a lot of practice. But once we have those in place, we are guaranteed the enjoyment of a happily-ever-after breastfeeding journey!

UNDERSTANDING AND DECIPHERING BREASTFEEDING PAINS (IN STOMACH, UTERUS, BREAST, NIPPLES)

*O*uch! No doubt, I know that many mamas, both new and seasoned, are not looking forward to this particular chapter. I mean, "Who wants to read a chapter basically about breast pains when they are the very reasons why most of us dread the words, "pregnancy and breastfeeding" even before we become mothers?" But you know what, mamas? We've got this like we always do!

I think now is the perfect time to let you know what happened during my last two breastfeeding experiences. Do you remember I said that I had a breast reduction surgery where my areolas were completely removed? Good! So, two years after my surgery, I had my second child. With no idea of what was in store for us, I began breastfeeding her at the time of birth. And then it happened! One week later, I was told that my baby wasn't gaining enough weight, so my midwife advised me to give her formula to supplement the little breast milk that she could get out of my breast. I felt quite devastated and inadequate knowing that my breast milk wasn't enough for my little one. During the process, I also suffered from blocked milk ducts since the milk could not come out as it should. Things got worse for me, and eventually, it led to mastitis. Though it was a time of pain, trials, and tribulations for me, I breastfed my baby for 5 years.

Now you would think that I would have figured it all out by the time my third baby came. Well, I also thought I knew it all. Immediately, I started pumping to ensure a good supply of milk for my baby. However, by the third day of breastfeeding, she was very fussy at the breast, and I knew she was not getting enough. Again, I had to supplement while breastfeeding my baby. I began to get very depressed as I really wanted to breast-feed my daughter. Come on, who wouldn't? At this point, I felt like a complete failure – the worst mother ever! My midwife was afraid of my mental state, so she referred me to a psychia-trist. Fortunately, by the time my baby was three months, I was getting better not just physically but mentally and emotionally. Quite an emotional story, isn't it? Interestingly, sharing this story with you right now makes me feel just like a super-mama! -Because you know? Even though I had to tandem feed my two youngest babies for several months while switching between breastfeeding and giving them formula, I still ended up victori-ous! I did not just win but also created a great and stronger bond between myself and my babies, and that's all that matters!

Hence, it is crucial to note that some of the breastfeeding pains and problems we will be analyzing in this chapter are unavoidable. But let's take a look at the brighter side; these pains have remedies! And you wouldn't even know how to apply those solutions until you gain an adequate understanding of the problem or the source of your pain. I hope that convinces you that this chapter is essential? Without further ado, let's get started!

CAUSES OF BREASTFEEDING PAINS

Before we dive right into the actual nursing issues that cause your breast to hurt, let's talk about those killer cramps in the early days of nursing! I don't know about other experienced mamas, but for me, the pain feels just like the worst menstrual cramps, and guess what? It gets worse with each baby! The lucky thing for us is that it only lasts for a few days. But what exactly is happening when you feel those cramps?

At that moment, the oxytocin - the hormone responsible for triggering milk production - is causing your uterus to shrink back to its standard size. However, it is pretty painful and uncomfortable. The cramps are a sign that your body is healing correctly from the delivery. It also decreases the risk of uterine bleeding. So, the next time you can experience those killer cramps, take it all out on the oxytocin hormone! Now that we have gotten that out of the way, let's focus on the other painful nursing condition.

BREAST ENGORGEMENT

Of course, we all wish that our breasts produce and get filled with a sufficient quantity of milk. However, when you wait longer to breastfeed your baby with that already supplied milk, either by skipping a breastfeeding session or not keeping to time, the situation becomes different. This excess fullness in your breasts increases your blood flow and makes the breast tissues swell. Ultimately, your breasts become hard, tight, lumpy, and painful. Those are primary signs that you are experiencing breast engorgement!

Now let's do a quick flashback; remember the very first moment your mature milk came in with increased supply? Remember that the first rush comes with pain, right? That's your first encounter with breast engorgement! The more engorged your breasts become, the more uncomfortable and painful the pain becomes. Your baby also gets affected by this. How? It becomes difficult for them to latch on to engorged breasts because the nipples tend to become flat.

Now, our first-time mamas might ask, "Is breast engorgement something that we have to deal with on a normal basis?" Not at all! Your breasts wouldn't get engorged if you emptied them frequently. How can you ensure that you drain your breast thoroughly? In the previous chapter, we already discussed how feeding the baby at appropriate intervals, maybe around 8 to 12 times in a complete day, can help ensure that you fully drain your breast milk. Yes! Being more frequent in feeding will surely help with the initial discomfort and eventually prevent engorgement.

Now, what if you feel that your milk suddenly comes in and your breast becomes full, but you can't feed your baby right away? - Maybe because you are at work or school? Not to worry, there are techniques you can use in preventing engorgement!

You can either try to pump or manually express your milk with your hands. Breast pumping is a topic we will soon explore. So let's wait and see. Now about hand expressing your milk, let's do a step-by-step analysis.

Start by holding onto your breast with your fingers underneath it and your thumb on top. Then gently but firmly press your thumb and fingers back against your chest. Next, roll your thumb and fingers against your chest wall and down toward your areola over and over. Doing this will surely help push the milk down your milk ducts.

Now we all know that there are times where you cannot help but experience breast engorgement. For instance, when I was at the grocery store, I heard a baby crying somewhere in the store; suddenly, I felt my breast become full and heavy with milk. I had only just got to the store, so there was no way I could trek back home to breastfeed my baby. Pumping or manually expressing my breast milk weren't reasonable options either. So, I had to struggle with the pain until I finished shopping. Viola! I get home with my engorged breasts but my baby finds it difficult to latch on. So, what decisions are we to consider in situations like that?

- First of all, you need to prepare ahead. Avoid wearing underwired bras and instead, go for wearing a correct-fitting breastfeeding bra. Such a bra will help you minimize the discomfort if you ever have to deal with breast engorgement.
- To make the swelling decrease, you can apply cold compresses to your breasts between feedings. It will even reduce tightness and pain around your breast.
- You can also try squeezing out a little amount of milk manually. This hand expression will help soften your areola and nipple, making it a lot easier for your baby to latch on.
- Just like cold compresses, applying warm compresses also works. You can also improvise by taking warm showers or leaning your breasts over warm water. All of this will make it easy to feed your baby.
- And of course! Massaging is an option that works great in milk flow.

Blocked Milk Ducts

In the first chapter, we learned about how the breast houses various milk ducts – those tubes transport milk after being produced in the milk glands to your nipple. Just like the way the pipes in your house get clogged if something gets stuck, the milk ducts can get blocked when you don't completely drain them. But the problem doesn't just stop at the blockage. The blocked milk ducts can, in turn, cause lumps in your breast. So, if you have ever seen somebody's breast skin red, that's the area where the node is. It is usually excruciating. In worse cases, the nipple can also have 8 to 9 openings blocked. This plugged opening just appears like a white dot on the end of the nipple.

What can you do when you experience a clogged milk duct? First, keep breastfeeding your baby from the breast that has a clogged vent. I know feeding your newborn from that breast can be challenging, but it can be very effective. You can also try placing the chin of your baby to point towards the lump area. Consider switching between different breastfeeding positions from cradle hold to football hold. Altering these positions might help ensure that all your milk ducts get entirely drained.

Also, as you feed your baby, gently massage the area of the pain lumps towards your nipple. Using warm compresses or warm flannels can help to make your milk flow more freely from the duct. Personally, what worked for me was that I would first pamper my breast with some warmth while in the shower, then hand-express my breast milk before finally pumping. All in all, I would recommend that you should see your doctor or a lactation consultant if the painful lump persists after two to three days.

Mastitis

Constant engorgement or an untreated blocked duct can lead to painful inflammation of your breast tissues. Inflammation is just one of the significant symptoms of mastitis. Apart from the soreness in the breast, you could also notice one red spot or streaks all over your breast. You might also experience flu-related symptoms like high temperature, fever, or chills. Now having mastitis isn't a death sentence but an infection that antibiotics can easily treat. If you find that you have mastitis, simply book an appointment with your doctor and get treated. Of course, we also have some remedies to share.

Continue breastfeeding your baby from the infected breast. No! Your baby wouldn't get infected at all! Though I must warn that continuous feeding on the affected breast will be pretty painful, but trust me, it can help clear up the infection. But if it is too hard or painful to feed your baby, express the milk manually through your hand or by pumping.

Surprisingly, proper positioning and latching are pretty crucial in preventing and treating mastitis. How? Suppose your baby is well-positioned and latched adequately. In that case, it becomes quick for her to empty your breast, eliminating chances of clogging or blockage. Most importantly, ensure that you get enough rest, especially after taking your antibiotics.

Cracked or Sore Nipples

No nursing mother's story is ever complete without them talking about nightmares of sore, cracked, and even blistered nipples. If you're currently struggling with intense soreness in your nipple, don't give up, mama, because you are not alone. It's only a phase; eventually, your nipples will heal, and they will be in a better condition than they were in the first place.

WHAT CAUSES SORENESS IN MY NIPPLES?

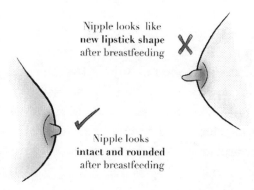

Nipple looks like **new lipstick shape** after breastfeeding

Nipple looks **intact and rounded** after breastfeeding

Poor latch

Judging from what we have learned from the last three chapters, even our newbie mamas would have guessed that would be the first point! The ultimate result of the poor latch is usually very uncomfortable and painful. Your nipples hurt so much as you are trying to breastfeed your baby. With time, they start looking squashed or blistered after you break the suction and bring it out from your baby's mouth. Ouch! See why we spend almost three chapters repeating the same thing! Now, what can you do to solve this problem? We have repeated these solutions multiple times, but it wouldn't hurt to do it one more time, right?

Learning how to latch your baby correctly is one of the best things you can do to help yourself and your baby. Like learning to drive, latching takes time and constant practice to become good at it. But if you keep working hard, you will quickly realize you get better with every single practice! And before you know it! You're already teaching other moms the secrets of the game!

Always remember that your baby's mouth should cover both your nipple and your areola. Her chin and nose should also be touching your breast as she feeds with her lips flanged outwards. For you to achieve a proper latch, you need to first be in the correct breastfeeding position. We've discussed four different holds, so take your time and pick out the ones that work best for you and your baby. In case you're still having trouble learning how to position and latch on your own, reach out to a seasoned mama, maybe your mum, or even your friend or seek professional help from a breastfeeding specialist or a lactation consultant.

NIPPLE SENSITIVITY

There is no escape for us regarding sensitive nipples. In fact, from my experience and my countless interactions with other moms, I think nipple sensitivity is a widespread complaint when we come in fresh.

How exactly does it feel? It's usually like you have pins and needles stabbing in your nipples. It can get quite intense when your baby begins to nurse. The fortunate thing is that it only lasts for about 30 seconds; that makes it easy to endure.

Another good news that might gladden your heart is that the intense sensitivity usually improves and perhaps disappears on its own by the time your baby is about a week old. Still, suppose you are like me, and you can't endure the sensitivity. In that case, you can use warm or cool compresses before and after breastfeeding your baby. An OTC pain reliever like acetaminophen may also do the magic of relieving discomfort.

Thrush

Does the name sound unfamiliar? Oh, it's just a fancy way of describing yeast infection in the nipple. Now there is no one who does not have yeast in their systems! Even Queen Beyonce does! And it is outstanding. But you see, the moment the yeast in our systems begins to overgrow, it poses many problems. But first, let's find out what could be responsible for causing yeast infection in the breasts?

Now you might have probably heard somebody somewhere say to you, "Make sure you wipe your nipples clean and dry after nursing your baby." Of course, it is a recognized way of maintaining personal hygiene. Still, that person is also trying to protect you from a yeast infection. A yeast infection may also occur when your iron level is deficient or when you are getting an antibiotic treatment.

Dear newbie mamas, I'm going to scare you a little bit here but keep in mind that we are just trying to learn as much as we can about these breastfeeding conditions. So, having a yeast infection means that you will have to deal with sore nipples, especially when you are nursing your baby. What's even worse

KIMBERLY NICOLE WHITTAKER

is that the pain, in this case, is usually on another level. The infection comes with sharp and stabbing pain. Though the skin of your breast may look smooth and shiny, you will also notice a pink or red rash around your nipples. Unfortunately, even the little one experiences the symptoms. He might also develop an oral thrush. The symptoms you are likely to notice are white dots or circles on the inside of your baby's lips and cheeks or maybe on the roof of his mouth. Sounds pretty painful, right?

I hope none of us get to experience this condition. But if life ends up happening like it usually does, ensure that you consult your doctor or midwife first to confirm the diagnosis. Then you can get a prescription for medication. Even if you are the only one experiencing the symptoms, your doctor would most likely advise and recommend that both you and your baby get treated. Getting treatment as early as possible is very important because things can go from bad to worse when you delay time. Now I know not every one of us can get immediate access to see a doctor; thus, you may consider going for a recommendation for an over-the-counter medication. Most women have recommended acidophilus supplements to be very helpful.

Remember that yeast infection could be because your iron levels are low? What does that tell us? It's simple: initiating a few dietary changes can also make a lot of difference! We have revealed how eating foods like oats, beef, lean meat, poultry, and so on can help supply you with a sufficient amount of iron, so make your choice!

Apart from your diet, you will also have to keep your nipple dry, especially after nursing your baby. You should do this because the yeast thrives on moisture, so if you don't give it that chance, it can't survive!

Painful Teething

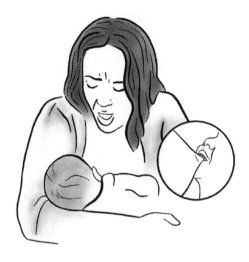

Have you ever wondered why many mamas stop breastfeeding the moment their babies start producing teeth? Well, we have the answer here. Now, around the 3rd or 4th month of birth, your baby began to feel her first milk teeth pushing through her gum. Along with this milestone, your baby also feels a kind of pressure. That uncomfortable pressure is what we refer to as teething. Your cutie would surely want to get relief from the discomfort, so she turns to her mom's nipples to get it. By biting and chewing on your nipple, your baby brings to settle and numb her gum. Quite a painful irony, isn't it?

Well, no matter how much we desire to be superheroes and save our babies from pain, getting our nipples bitten and chewed is not an option for consideration. To fix the effects of her painful teething, you can give your baby a teething toy or frozen wet washcloth just before you start to breastfeed. These may help relieve the discomfort, making it more convenient for her onto latch your nipple and settle into the feeding.

If your baby is still gnawing on your breast, immediately break the suction and give her the teething toy or frozen wet washcloth again. You can also try to use gentle words like, "don't bite." Now I know your baby doesn't understand the art of speech but guess what? You have something even more potent and better - the emotional intimacy you share with your child. Take advantage of it and help your baby understand action and consequence!

Nipple Blanching and Vasospasm

Trust me, these conditions are just as problematic as their names sound. Let's start with nipple blanching. When your baby gets so excited about feeding, he may bore down a little too hard on your nipples. By doing this, it is most likely that your nipple would pop out of his mouth looking almost like the tip of your lipstick -- all whitened and in a funny shape! That's how nipple blanching occurs.

Now about nipple vasospasm; you know the nipple is already in a compressed condition from the blanching. That tight state results in vasospasm, in which the blood vessels around your nipple contract abnormally. I don't have to tell us how extremely painful that can be, right?

For this reason, it is much better when you detect the problem early at the stage of blanching. That way, you only have to correct the way you position and latch your baby either on your own or with professional help. However, the moment it results in vasospasm, treatment can be more challenging. In most cases, the vasospasm tends to become worse when you're cold. Try everything warm, warm compresses, and warm wash-cloths before nursing to breastfeeding in warm environments and wearing warm clothes. You can also try massaging your areola with olive oil to stretch the blood vessels a little! No matter how much you love caffeine, you should avoid it because it will make the problem worse.

. . .

PAIN FROM PUMPING Equipment

I have mentioned several times already that pumping is a breastfeeding technique that requires concentration, practice, and patience to master. Many of us mamas have little or no idea about using the pump correctly and effectively, but we go with the flow! As such, you might end up pumping your breast over-vigorously with a high suction setting. It could also be that you position the flange incorrectly or even use the wrong flange size. All of these could be pretty bad for your nipple, leaving them all sore and painful.

Though we have a whole chapter dedicated to helping us learn about pumping, let's do a quick overview on how you can prevent pain from pumping equipment. Firstly, make sure you are setting out for the pumping game with the correct flange size and suction settings on your pump. How do you know if it is the right one? Your nipple should be in the center of the pump flange tunnel. Also, your nipple should be moving freely throughout the pumping process without a more considerable amount of your areola sucking into the flange tunnel.

HOW CAN I RELIEVE MY CRACKED AND SORE NIPPLES WHEN BREASTFEEDING?

In addition to the problems, we have examined some breast-feeding solutions. Here are a few tips that can be of help.

- You can soothe the sore nipples by getting a recommended cream from your doctor. An ultra-pure lanolin cream is a go-to option that works for many mamas, including myself. So, all you have to do is gently pat a small portion of lanolin to your nipple and areola. It can also help with the dry breast skin around that area. You can also apply frozen hydrogel pads. Trust me; that nipple-dressing can cool your breastfeeding pain like magic.

- If you can't access any of the two options mentioned above, you could gently apply a few drops of your breast milk around your sore nipples. At least with that, you wouldn't have to remove anything to feed your baby. Or you could try mixing your breast milk with a little bit of vitamin D ointment before applying it before every breastfeeding session. That method did magic in relieving nipple soreness during my three breastfeeding experiences. Essentially, all three lubricating elements provide a moisture barrier that will help limit your breast skin's moisture.

- Sometimes, the only non-medicated drug you need is patience and endurance! For some of these breastfeeding pains, the soreness usually numbs down when our body begins to get used to breastfeeding and when our baby learns to latch early and efficiently. That would probably take about a few days or weeks.

- Whether your nipple is infected or sore, ensure that you wipe gently and carefully, especially after nursing your baby. You can consider using water-moistened cotton wool to wipe and remove any debris that could lead to infection or cause further harm. It's soft and less painful.

- If soaking up milk leakage, you should never forget to regularly change your disposable or washable nursing pads.

- We have said way too much about latching, but you get a deeper and more proper latch if you try different breastfeeding positions. Beyond that, exploring other places like the laid-back, cross-cradle, or football position can remove the pressure off the most painful areas of your breast.

- Have you ever heard of breast shields? Mind you, they are not nipple shields! Breast shields are dome-shaped shields that you can use in between feedings to prevent your sore nipples from rubbing against clothing. That way, they can help them heal faster.
- Every time you break suction when your baby completes breastfeeding, ensure that you do it gently. You could slip your finger into the side of your baby's mouth or in-between the gums, then make a quarter turn with your finger to break the suction.
- To cap it all, get plenty of rest and stay happy!

Leaky Breasts

Leaking doesn't cause breastfeeding pain, but it can pose a problem. Imagine being out with your friends or even during a presentation at work. All of a sudden, you soaked through your blouse! It could be very embarrassing, right? Unfortunately, leaky breasts are something we mamas have to deal with, especially in the first weeks of breastfeeding. Often, it is usually stimulated unexpectedly by the let-down reflex. Remember when I said my milk suddenly came in when I heard any baby crying at the grocery store? That's the effect of the let-down reflex. We can also blame it on the oxytocin hormones since they help you produce milk and create an emotional bond with your baby. How sweet, right? Well, not until it turns on the milk-making sprinklers when you least expect it.

Since you might have to keep dealing with leaky breasts for at least the first six weeks of breastfeeding or so, you might want to consider wearing disposable or washable nursing pads inside your bra both during the day and at night to soak up the leakage and protect your shirt at all times!

And it's a wrap! Just like that! It wasn't that bad, was it? Now that we have gained an in-depth understanding of how we can solve our breastfeeding problems when they arise, we are in a better position to be the best version of ourselves for our babies. Nevertheless, it is always advisable to seek the advice and help of your doctor, especially when problems arise. Early treatment is the best! As you struggle and conquer all these problems, ensure that you take only the appropriate therapies. Keep doing that as you enjoy building that unique, intimate bond with your newborn during breastfeeding!

GIVEAWAY

A FREE GIFT FOR OUR READERS!

Five adaptable recipes you can download and start your breastfeeding journey off on a delicious foot!! Visit this link

KimberlyNicoleWhittaker.com

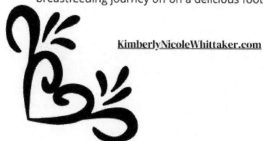

NORMAL TO OVERACTIVE LETDOWN

With all the latching issues, sore nipples, and milk flow problems that we have discussed so far, I'm sure many of us, especially the first-time mamas, would agree that the journey of breastfeeding can be very tricky and not-as-easy-as-it-looks. Indeed, it is! But trust me, the feeling every time your baby looks at you as you breastfeed her is like love at first sight; it makes everything else fade away. Now enough of the motivation; I just needed to get us gingered up for this chapter! I sure hope we are!

Now, 'the letdown reflex" is a phrase we have used several times in the previous chapters. Perhaps you might have guessed its meaning, but it is one of those actions that can make it easier to breastfeed your baby. So, what exactly is the letdown reflex?

Now, from the top. When the tiny nerves in your nipple get stimulated by your baby sucking your breast, or you hear her cry. Or maybe just the mere thought of your newborn; those nerves send signals to your brain. Thus, this causes the two hormones, prolactin, and oxytocin to be released. I guess that by now, these two names would be familiar terms in your vocabulary. Anyways, as we have said before, prolactin acts on the milk-making glands (alveoli) in your breast, which leads to milk production. The oxytocin hormone takes up the job from there and causes the milk to be released and let down into the milk ducts, then to the outer openings in your nipple, and finally to your baby's mouth!

I hope you didn't miss that part where we said, "The milk is then letdown." That is it! In short, we can conclude that the letdown reflex helps make breast milk available to your baby. Now you see why I said it is one of those actions that make breastfeeding easier for you and your baby. Surprisingly, the letdown reflex usually happens more than once during a breast-feeding session. However, most of us tend only to notice the first one. Those other letdowns typically occur in response to changes in your baby's suckling.

We've already made it clear that the letdown reflex can be triggered when you see or hear your baby or perhaps when you think about them. Well, the power to start the nerves is not only limited to your baby. Touching your breast and nipple area with your fingers can also impact your letdown. This reaction explains how you can hand-express milk to your baby. Also, the use of a breast pump can stimulate the letdown reflex. For me and perhaps for some mamas reading this, our emotional state impacts our letdown reflex. For instance, if I'm incredibly anxious, angry, tired, or in pain, the letdown may take longer than usual.

Essentially, we cannot overemphasize that breastfeeding, being a mighty process, is unique for every mama. In the same way, the letdown reflex is different for every mother. What do I mean? Let's take a few steps back. Do you remember that in the first few days of your birth, some mothers get an increase in their breast milk supply very quickly while others don't? Good! But with time, we all know the other mother's milk supply will eventually adjust to the baby's needs.

Now that we have re-established that, you must understand

that letdown comes easily, naturally, and in moderation for some mamas when this increase in milk supply occurs. But for some of us, getting the milk to flow can be very difficult and slow. It could also be swift and forceful! Before we get into details about the quiet, regular, and fast modes of a letdown, each of us, especially the newbie mamas, must familiarize ourselves with the signs to expect when we are about to experience the action itself. But why is that important? It can help you determine whether your reflex is normal, slow, or overactive!

How do **I know when I have a letdown?**

Well, we, mamas, experience different kinds of sensations when the letdown occurs. In most cases, the feelings are always in or around your breasts. Let's examine a few of them;

- You may feel an intense tingling sensation, most likely from under your arm, and then it moves slowly across and down your breast. It's like pins and needles are pinching you from within your breast.
- Your breast might also feel full and heavy.
- Oh! You shouldn't be surprised if milk begins to drip or even shoot out from your other breast. It's a letdown sign!
- Apart from within or around your breast, you might also experience intense cramping in your uterus as you let down, especially if it's not your first baby. Usually, it goes away after the early days of your baby's birth. But why does this have to happen in the first place? In the previous chapter, I had asked you to blame the cramps on the oxytocin hormone. Many mamas, including experienced ones like myself, might not know that breastfeeding helps your uterus quickly return to its standard size. Wait! What have all

these got to do with the letdown reflex? Well, mamas, in letting down your milk, the hormone-in-charge, oxytocin, also causes your uterus to contract gradually. Do you see the connection now?

Please, note that these sensations can develop immediately after birth for some mamas. Still, for others, the timing could be several weeks after they have started breastfeeding. Some mamas may not even feel their milk flow from their ducts to their nipples. Remember what we have always said? Every stage of the breastfeeding journey is different for every mama!

HOW CAN I QUICKLY GET MY LETDOWN TO OCCUR WHEN FEEDING OR EXPRESSING?

Like we stated earlier, letdown does not come relatively easy and natural for some of us mamas. But not to worry! We've got your back. Here are some ideas for your letdown process.

- Relax: Now you might be thinking, "Kim, how can I be calm and relaxed when my milk flow is slow for my baby? I understand how you feel but always remember that your stress has a way of inhibiting your letdown. So, while you are feeding your baby or trying to hand-express your milk, Take slow and deep breaths. Breastfeeding is thirsty work, so it might also be helpful to have a warm drink first, or you can keep a glass of water handy. You can consider the option of pampering your breast with some warmth, be it taking a warm shower or simply putting a friendly face washer on your breast before you start breastfeeding.
- Since we are already familiar with all these early cues that your baby will exhibit to show hunger, we should

ensure that we feed our babies immediately when we notice those signs. It will make a whole lot of difference in improving your letdown reflex.

- To encourage your letdown, you can gently massage your breasts. Now there is a trick to doing it efficiently. Stroke your breast towards the nipple with the web of your hand or using the edge of a finger. Then you gently roll your nipple between two of your fingers. Feels good, right? Aside from massaging your breast by yourself, you can also get your partner or support person to give you a gentle back and shoulder massage.

- Also, looking at your baby as you breastfeed her helps get the job done. You might not understand how exactly this is supposed to work but trust me, it works! When you are trying to express your milk on the hand, three secret tips can work for you. The easiest way is to hand express while your baby is near you. But when you are away from your baby, you could think about your baby – her smile and his cute looks. The last option is to express the milk while looking at a photo of your little one.

- Feeding your baby in private can also be a helpful tool. I know some mothers who feel like they are under pressure when anyone watches them breastfeed their baby. Now breastfeeding or expressing in private can work both ways. You wouldn't deal with any pressure, and your baby might enjoy the solitude more, thus allowing him to focus better.

- Doing a lean-forward position may also work. What you have to do is to lean forward and let your breast hang free from any clothing. So, you shake your breasts from side to side vigorously. Now, this

shouldn't be painful. The only thing that you should
be feeling is the weight of your breast moving.

DO I PRODUCE DIFFERENT TYPES OF MILK DURING MY LETDOWN?

Okay! This question is something we need to address real quick before we proceed! Dearest first-time and experienced mamas, have you ever been told that your breast milk comes in two types? The foremilk and hindmilk, right? Well, that isn't wholly true. Let's break down how the process occurs.

When your letdown reflex begins operation, it facilitates the gradual dislodgment of the fat globules in your breast from their dwelling through the milk ducts. Now keep the word 'gradual' in mind as we continue. So, the longer the breast-feeding session, the more the fat globules are forced out. Now, what does this mean? As your feeding progresses, the higher the fat content in your breast milk becomes.

Now, how do the foremilk and hindmilk come into place in all of these? So, the foremilk refers to the milk at the beginning of the feeding sessions. It is the waterier and lactose-rich component of breast milk. The hindmilk, on the other hand, is the milk at the end of the feeding session. This one offers more satiety to your baby because it is creamy and fat-rich. What you must understand is that there is no sharp distinction between these two milk types. They are just terms to identify the gradual changes in fat content at that stage of milk ejection. To under-stand better, let's use an illustration! Think about when you turn on the tap for a desirable or warm shower. You know the first water you get may not be hot but cold. But gradually, it gives you precisely what you want, which is hot water!

This process is what happens as your milk becomes available for your baby. At the very beginning, the fat content in breast milk isn't that high. However, as the breast begins to empty, the fat content increases. So, if you are perhaps convinced that your milk in your breast can transform at an arbitrary point to start producing hindmilk first instead of foremilk, then you need to discard that thought!

On this note, I must remind you that this is why we said in the previous chapter that you shouldn't switch sides when actively breastfeeding your baby. Instead, you should always allow your baby to drain your first breast before offering the second one. Now that we have cleared that misconception, let's move on!

OVERACTIVE LETDOWN

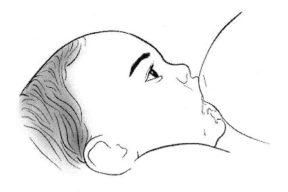

Usually, people save the best for the last, but we've saved the most complicated type of letdown for the final in today's chapter! Our biggest fear as mothers is usually not producing enough milk for our baby. Well, then permit me to ask, "How then do we cope when the milk supply increases to the point that it begins to affect our babies negatively? That's a tough one.

I can't give the correct answer because my breastfeeding

challenge was mainly due to insufficient milk supply. Anyways, one of my closest friends suffered the direct opposite of my problem - an overactive or what some people call "forceful letdown"!

Surprisingly, it wasn't even her first baby. Since she was already experienced, this beautiful mama was sure that her breastfeeding journey would be smooth and easy. Unfortunately, things turned out differently right from the first few days of her nursing her baby. Her baby boy kept choking, coughing, and pulling off every time she attempted to breast-feed him. Now it wasn't that the boy was satisfied. He exhibited all the necessary hunger cues we've talked about earlier, from being fussy to even crying. To make things worse, the mama was also sore. Her lactation consultant finally helped diagnose the problem to be a case of an overactive letdown, and then she went on to suggest solutions.

Nevertheless, I saw my friend go through so much, from constantly being messy and suffering public leaking humilia-tions to the never-ending worries about her baby's gas. But guess what? Her mindset to succeed at breastfeeding even with all the challenges inspired me, and I'm sure it will do the same to you! Others were looking at her and thinking, "Oh! What a nightmare!" But for my friend, every moment was worth it!

Now the truth is that it was not an easy journey at all, but she won! Her newborn is already all grown up and in kinder-garten. And oh! He is so cute; he thinks his mum is the best thing in the world after chocolate! If you're in this same boat of an overactive letdown, you have nothing to worry about because together, you and I will go over the many techniques you can use to get your letdown reflex under control!

But first, we need to understand what we are dealing with here. What exactly happens when you say some mamas have a fast letdown? By being fast, it means your letdown reflex is on overdrive! Your breast milk rushes through your milk ducts and out the nipple a little too fast and hard at letdown. Imagine how fast water spurts out from a firefighter's hose! Like a flash, right? Now, what would happen if you tried drinking water straight from a firefighter's hose? Too much to handle, isn't it? Precisely that's why the babies in this condition tend to cough and choke. In most cases, an overactive letdown has connections with having an oversupply of milk.

WHY IS MY LETDOWN OVERACTIVE?

If you were following along very keenly, you would observe that I said something about the connection between overactive letdown and milk oversupply. Frequently, an overactive letdown reflex occurs due to an overload of milk. Well, a lactation consultant might call it "hyper-lactation." In plain English, this means that your breasts produce more than enough milk.

In the first six weeks of your baby's birth, especially during the "new mommy engorgement phase," your breast milk production is primarily controlled by your hormones (prolactin and oxytocin) instead of your baby's actual intake rate. So, it is a pretty common thing for most mamas' bodies to take the job too seriously and then overdo the production.

Though we said that an oversupply of milk often causes an overactive letdown, this is not always the reason in all cases. It could also occur when you take extra-long intervals in-between your breastfeeding sessions. So, the longer you delay the breast-feeds, the more the milk is produced and stored in the breast, leading to increased pressure, making the letdown spurt like a fire hose!

Furthermore, it could be because your baby has difficulty latching. This condition is potentially resulted in when your baby has a tongue-tie. We will go into details about this condition in the next chapter so stick with me! But at this point, you should keep in mind that tongue-tied babies usually have difficulty latching.

HOW CAN I EVEN BE SURE THAT I HAVE AN OVERACTIVE LETDOWN?

My friend had no idea that she was having an overactive letdown until she went to see a lactation consultant. I know many mamas in the same condition have the same problem, and maybe they might not have the chance to see a lactation consultant. So to make thing much easier for you, we have gathered some common signs you can look out for to be sure if you are having an overactive letdown;

- Your baby chokes frequently and coughs.
- Her latches are primarily poor and shallow. It can also be that your baby constantly pulls away and resists your breast while crying, or she clamps down on your nipple. These are some coping mechanisms that babies use when they are dealing with an overactive letdown.
- In one of the previous chapters, we learned that one primary way to identify a bad latch is that your baby makes clicking sounds and not gulping sounds. It could also signal an overactive letdown, especially if you notice that the milk dribbles through the side of her mouth.
- When your baby starts to react with excessive gas by constantly farting, belching, hiccupping, or spitting up, then it could be because you are having an overactive letdown. So, what's the relationship between the excess gas and your overactive letdown? Your baby being gassy or colicky maybe because she is consuming excess foremilk and not enough

hindmilk – a situation that is most common with an overactive letdown. Research has proven that babies who receive too much foremilk tend to suffer from hunger, colic, and excess gas because foremilk digests too quickly.

- Now away from your breast and milk, let's see your baby's diapers! You may suspect an overactive letdown when your baby's poop is usually foamy and green. This particular sign shows your baby is getting excess foremilk which is rich in lactose.
- The signs can also be from you. You will notice your nipples getting sore and your breasts leaking more often than expected.

HOW CAN I OVERCOME MY LETDOWN CHALLENGES?

- **Try laid-back breastfeeding positions:** Do we have to do a flashback, or we all remember what this breastfeeding position is? Well, a quick reminder; the laid-back pose also referred to as 'biological nurturing,' involves you resting back with your baby facing your belly. All she has to do is to reach for your breast and latch on. We said that the laid-back is a great breastfeeding position for mamas with overactive letdown reactions and gassy babies. The reason is that breastfeeding in this position allows you to take advantage of gravity to slow milk flow into your baby's mouth. It's also pretty comfortable! At night, you could try the side-lying position. By doing that, the excess milk can quickly dribble out of the breast and perhaps through the side of your baby's mouth this way.

- When you notice your baby let go of your breast because of the fast flow of milk, resist the temptation to hold the back of his head to force him to latch onto the breast! You will only make your baby's agitation worse by doing that! By letting go of the breast, your baby is trying to protect his airways so he can breathe. So, allow him to enjoy his break!

- As much as possible, you should avoid taking long time intervals in between your breastfeeding sessions. Instead, you should try feeding your baby frequently and on-demand too! Doing this will help you reduce faster milk flow due to the increased pressure of milk within the breast. It even eliminates chances of painful engorgement.

- This particular tip is a bit tricky. But believe me, it is very effective. So, studies have shown that many babies struggle the most with the fast flow of milk during the actual milk letdown. We've already learned a bit earlier that the first letdown usually takes place 30 seconds to a few minutes into the feeding. Here is the trick! You're already familiar with the letdown signs. Good! So, what you do is that the moment you begin to feel those signs, you let your baby off your breast and then catch the forceful milk in a breast milk bag or towel! Once you think that the first letdown is complete, you re-latch the baby and feed him. Now, the goal is after catching the forceful milk that tends to rush in with the letdown reflex, the flow wouldn't be that hard or fast.

Dear mamas, whether you are having a slow letdown or a fast one, giving up should not be an option! The most crucial lesson we should all take from this chapter is that it gets better! Both for you and your baby! As your newborn grows, he begins to cope and even enjoy your overactive letdown! This statement might be hard to believe, especially if you are dealing with an overactive letdown. But it's the truth! For now, what you do is internalize and materialize all the tips mentioned above to help you get through those frustrating early days or weeks after delivery. Here is a big shout-out to every mama who struggles with their letdown reflex yet still makes breastfeeding look so effortlessly!

IS IT A TIE?

*A*s I promised earlier, this chapter is going to be all about tongue-tie. What does it mean? How is it caused? The effects it has as well as the likely treatment approaches for the condition? Of course, there would be so much more in-between as we go through each of these areas. Let's start with a quick question; would you be shocked if I told you that your tongue takes up the most significant part of your mouth? I bet a lot of mamas would be!

Anyways, it only sounds logical to say that the tongue does most of the job to enhance your baby's ability to feed. Sounds confusing? You know what? Let's try this again.

So, the tongue is the most important of your organs housed within your mouth and that of your baby. Why is that? Well, without her tongue, your baby can't latch onto your breast correctly enough to trigger the letdown reflex and then draw out breast milk. If you don't believe me, then try observing keenly the next time your baby gets ready to latch. You would notice that the first thing she would do is extend her tongue out to take the nipple and some surrounding areolae into her mouth. Even as she drinks the milk from your breast, it is also with her tongue that she can form a good seal around the latch.

All of these sound good and easy. However, your baby's tongue has to be capable of reaching every part of her mouth before she can do all these latching-related functions effectively. Even you, her mama, need to be able to move your tongue in a full range of motion to be able to swallow food and even speak. Let's try this together; stretch your tongue out, then move it sideways both to the left and right, then upwards and downwards. That was way too easy for you. Well, some babies are not able to move their tongues in such a full range of motion.

Technically, this inability is because the body is born with a condition called 'Ankyloglossia.' Too hard to spell and pronounce. Well, let's save ourselves the trouble and stick to calling it 'a tongue-tie'. Yes, that's more like it! Just like the name implies, a tongue-tie ties your baby's tongue. Now, please stick with me and pay immense attention as we go on. In your baby's mouth, you would see a cord of tissue that connects the underside of her tongue to the bottom of the mouth. That band of tissue is called the lingual frenulum.

Under normal circumstances, the cord is long and flexible. However, when a baby is born with a tongue-tie, the frenulum is too short or too tight and thick. Having either of these two situations may inhibit the flexible movement of your baby's tongue. In the more complicated cases, the frenulum may be attached quite near the tip of her tongue. As such, the little one is unable to stick out her tongue past her gums.

At this point, I must emphasize that having a tongue-tie is a relatively common condition because studies have shown that about 4% to 11% of all newborns are born with it. So dear mamas, you don't have to be scared if your baby has a tongue-tie. I promise it's not a chronic illness. Now, I know some pregnant mamas-to-be might also be thinking, "Oh, what are the causes of a tongue-tie so that we can avoid them to ensure that our babies don't get it?" I do wish I had the answer to that question, but sadly I don't. The factors responsible for a tongue-tied are mainly unknown. As of now, the only discovery that researchers have been able to verify is that sometimes a tongue-tie can be caused by specific genetic factors. That is, if it runs in the family, then there is a reasonable probability that your baby may also develop it. Studies have discovered that a tongue-tie is more common in baby boys than girls. Now keep in mind, this doesn't mean that it cannot affect anyone. It just implies that more cases of this condition came from boys than girls. Are we clear?

In addition, from my research and the conversations I have had with mamas whose babies were tongue-tied, I discovered that doctors don't always check for the condition. Besides, it is not always easy to notice, especially during the first few hours and days after delivery. Thus, it could be that you and your baby sign out from the hospital, but neither you nor the medical professionals have any clue about the condition. Now, that's not a big deal because even if your child's doctor does not discover the situation until later, he can still make corrections with excellent results. Nevertheless, you have to be very observant to actually notice it. Here are some signs you should be the lookout for if you suspect that your baby has a tongue-tie;

- Your baby has great trouble sticking his tongue beyond his lower front teeth.
- She finds it difficult to lift her tongue to the upper teeth or move the tongue from side to side.
- Your baby's tongue looks like it's heart-shaped or notched when she sticks it out.

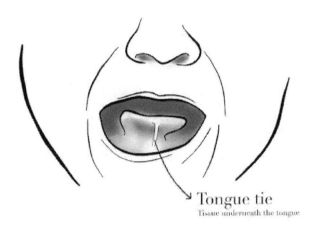

Tongue tie
Tissue underneath the tongue

WHAT COMPLICATIONS CAN A TONGUE-TIE CAUSE?

Firstly, we must understand that tongue-tie might not be an issue for both the baby and his mama. However, when the case is different, we can have some complications that go both ways for you and your baby. Let's start with your baby!

INTERFERES with your baby's feeding ability: We already know that for your nursing session to be practical, your baby must be able to extend his or her tongue over the lower gum to suck. However, since a tongue-tied baby might not be able to move his tongue beyond his lower teeth or in a full range of motion, he might be unable to suck correctly on the nipple. Hence, the newborn might employ the next available option to chew the nipple with his teeth. Apart from the fact that this action would be harrowing for the mother, the baby is most likely not to gulp down a sufficient amount of milk. Instead, you will notice the milk pouring out through the sides of his mouth.

. . .

Poor nutrition: Ultimately, your tongue-tied baby's inability to latch on and breastfeed effectively can end up affecting his food intake negatively. If that happens, you would see the signs. Your baby's weight may not increase as it should. Also, the newborn might not be producing the expected number of dirty diapers, and the few are likely to be filled with foamy and green poop. Of course, all of these are signs that will help you know that something is undoubtedly wrong.

Difficulty in speech and other oral activities: Now, I know this isn't related to breastfeeding. However, they are complications that may arise in the future if your baby's tongue-tie is left untreated. So how exactly does the condition affect your baby's speech pattern? Simply put, a tongue-tie interferes with your baby's ability to pronounce words, especially when it comes to sounds like" "d," "z," "s," "r," and "l." It could also impact his other oral activities. For instance, activities such as licking an ice cream cone, licking off food bits off his lips, kissing, or even playing a wind instrument, etc., might not be easy tasks for your baby.

Your baby's dental health may also be at risk if the tongue-tie is left untreated as she grows up. Oral problems such as tooth decay and swollen and irritated gum are likely to come up. Interestingly, a tongue-tie can be the reason for your baby having a gap between the lower two front teeth.

Somehow, I think the last one would make the baby look cuter. I was kidding, though! Now, how does my baby's tongue-tie affect you as a breastfeeding mother?

Painful breast problems: I'm sure you haven't forgotten what we said earlier about a tongue-tied baby being more likely to chew rather than suck on his mama's nipple. We don't need any sage to tell us how bad and painful that can be. Apart from chewing, a tongue-tie can indirectly increase other painful breast problems such as breast engorgement, significant nipple pain, plugged milk ducts, and mastitis. Drawing from the lessons we have learned so far, you would acknowledge that all of the problems mentioned above have the exact root cause, which is the inability of your baby to empty the breasts of the breast milk.

DECREASE IN BREAST MILK SUPPLY: This is that point where we press the remote to do a little flashback. So, do we remember that a few chapters ago, we analyzed how milk production in the breast operates based on a demand and supply process? That is, the more your baby can feed on demand, the more your milk-making glands would be encouraged to reproduce and re-supply enough milk to meet your baby's previous intake. However, when the demand level is reduced and low, the same happens with the breast supply. So basically, when your baby cannot drain the breast of the already supplied breast milk, the milk-making glands do not get the signal to reproduce.

EMOTIONAL STRESS: All of the aforementioned painful breast-feeding problems can be very frustrating. Wait, let me rephrase that they ARE very disappointing, especially for first-time mothers. Having a tongue-tied baby requires you to be resilient and focused. Unless you are determined, there is a high possibility that it can lower your breastfeeding confidence. And we don't want that happening, do we?

EARLY WEANING: We cannot afford to see our little ones in pain. In the same way, there is a limit to the amount of pain we can tolerate. Due to this reason, many mamas who find themselves in this situation resort to weaning their babies quite early. So, they introduce their babies to formulas and solids quickly with the hope that things would get better for both of them.

HOW CAN I HELP MY TONGUE-TIED BABY BREASTFEED?

Having evaluated your baby's condition using the signs mentioned above, the first thing to do once you discover or suspect that your baby has a tongue-tie is to contact your doctor, midwife, or lactation consultant and fix an appointment.

This professional doctor would perform a more credible diagnosis and refer you and your baby for proper treatment. Two things are likely to happen. Firstly, your doctor or lactation consultant may recommend correcting the state of your baby's tongue straight away. In some cases, doctors manage to discover the condition. Hence, he administers the correction before discharging you and newborns. But what are these correction methods? We will get to know all about them in a bit but first, let's find out the second approach your doctor is likely to take.

In some cases, your doctor or lactation consultant may want to adopt a wait-and-see approach. That is, there is no special treatment. Based on the hypothesis, your doctor might conclude that the short, tight, or thick band of tissue will loosen over time. Of course, that's what we need to get your baby to start latching properly and feeding effectively.

You know I like saving the most complicated for the last, right? Great! A quick warning, though; the other recommended treatment for rectifying your baby's tongue-tie is quite a controversial one. But why is that? It involves surgery! Did I hear somebody say, 'Oh no!' See, that's why I said it's controversial. But honestly, this surgical procedure isn't all that serious.

However, no matter how small, surgery is always considered a sensitive topic in any part of the world.

Nevertheless, a tongue-tie is treatable with two surgical procedures. The choice of treatment approach depends solely on your baby's age and the symptoms and severity of the condition. Remember we said the tie could be short, thick, or tight. Also, you could tie it so close to the tip of the tongue. Now you might not know this, but each of these cases differs in severity. Okay, let's see what these two surgical procedures are.

FRENOTOMY

Frenotomy is a simple surgical procedure that involves the doctor examining your baby's lingual frenulum and then using a laser or sterile scissors to snip the frenulum free. Ouch! What comes next? Intense bleeding, isn't it? Surprisingly, it is only likely to have only a drop or two drops of blood; even that depends on whether any bleeding occurs, usually in rare cases. The lack of bleeding is because there are few nerve endings or blood vessels in the lingual frenulum. Just like the blood, your baby will only have to deal with very minimal discomfort and pain.

You can think of it as going to the doctor's office to examine and clean up your wound. A frenotomy is a procedure that can be done relatively quickly in your doctor's office or perhaps in the hospital nursery. Some of the mamas and doctors I spoke to revealed that you could do this with or without anesthesia. Imagine that! You can breastfeed your baby immediately after. Now I said something about this procedure is controversial, right?

Though we can all conclude that the frenotomy is a low-risk procedure, some people question if complications like bleeding, infection, and damages to the tongue and salivary glands, and even the regrowth of the tight tongue tie, might arise. But ultimately, the decision to release the tongue tie is between the baby's mom and the pediatrician.

FRENULOPLASTY

Now we have something a little bit more extensive than the frenotomy - a frenuloplasty. This surgical procedure can be a recommended option if your baby's lingual frenulum is too thick for a frenotomy or perhaps if it requires extra repair. The processes in a frenuloplasty are usually the direct opposite of the frenulum.

So, your baby's surgery would be done under general anesthesia with surgical tools in this case. After the doctor frees the frenulum tissue, the wound will then be closed with sutures. Of course, we don't do this with the frenotomy. Nonetheless, the sutures are absorbed on their own as your baby's tongue gets healed. Due to the extensiveness of the surgery, your baby might have to deal with scarring in the future. Fortunately, there is a way out! Simply exercising the tongue primarily through stretching can reduce the chances of scarring and even enhance the overall tongue movement. Just like the frenotomy, people also have a controversial opinion about a frenuloplasty. This controversy is prominent because of possible complications such as bleeding, infection, or damage to the tongue or salivary glands. Usually, these occurrences are rare.

That's it about the two surgical treatments that would likely be recommended by your doctor when it comes to treating a tongue-tie. However, the most important lesson I want us to take from this chapter is that the treatment of a tongue tie is possible even if it poses a massive challenge to your breast-feeding journey. Another thing you must understand as a mama with a tongue-tied baby is that complete treatment requires an excellent team effort. So it doesn't just involve your child's pediatrician or doctors; you can also see a lactation consultant, speech pathologist, and even an occupational therapist for additional help and support. Treating your baby's tongue-tie may not solve all your breastfeeding problems but believe me and the countless proven studies, it has high capabilities of resolving and improving the situation. So, cheers to a more prosperous, effective, and less painful breastfeeding session that lasts for a greater length of time!

NIPPLE CONFUSION AND BREAST REFUSAL

*N*ipple confusion and breast refusal were terms that I never really understood until my last two breast-feeding experiences. While breastfeeding my first child, my doctor and midwife let me know that the way to prevent such reactions from my baby was to avoid introducing him to any artificial nipples, especially during the first few weeks when he was trying to perfect his perfect breastfeeding and sealing skills. At that time, I did not bother to ask in-depth questions because I considered the advice unnecessary since I was more than ready to breastfeed my son exclusively for as long as possible.

I wished I had listened when I had the chance to learn freely and without pressure. After my surgery, my breastfeeding experiences somewhat surrounded these concepts. Even though I had a complete desire to breastfeed my baby without any artificial nipple, I could not do that since I had to give my baby instant formula and other supplements. By feeding my baby with bottles of formulas as early as the first few days of birth, you could say that the two of them exhibiting symptoms of nipple confusion and breast refusal were almost pre-programmed. But mind you, I did not know what was happening at first. Having been told that my second child needed more nourishment, I started feeding her soy formula while trying to pump and breastfeed her with as much breast milk as I could deliver. Another thing to note is that I did not have enough time to research the problem, so I did not know what to expect. I did not realize that I needed to learn more.

Gradually, I noticed that my baby girl would feed comfortably well on a bottle, but when I tried to breastfeed her, she pulled after only a few minutes. Guess what was even worse about the situation? Her grunting and arching mainly characterized those short periods of perhaps 8 to 12 minutes of nursing. It was so frustrating for me! At one point, I started feeling like my baby hated me!

I did not fully realize that my baby's actions were natural reactions to his feeding circumstances. It was a long journey, but with the help of my midwife, my babies became very efficient feeders, both with the bottle and the breast. Now, I know that some mamas would be thinking, "That is what my dream goal is." Well, I have got you as usual!

This chapter will uncover the different actions you need to either discard or develop to achieve this goal! A little disclaimer, though! I am fully aware that your breastfeeding challenges are not the same as mine, or perhaps they are, but either way, this chapter is going to be as extensive as possible so that no mama feels left out! It is a promise! So, if you are ready to do it, shall we begin?

As a mother, positioning your baby and getting him to latch correctly is quite the job. Well, you should also keep in mind that the actions of latching on and drawing out milk from your breast are also hard work for your baby, which is why we said before that, after birth, your baby needs time to learn and perfect these breastfeeding skills. You should not be amazed to know that these latching skills are not inborn for a newborn, unlike most of us previously assumed.

Now, let us take a pause here to do a quick rundown of the processes involved in transporting milk from the milk-making glands in your breast to the belly of your baby. Did I hear some mamas complaining that we have already discussed this quite a few times in the preceding chapters? We need it again, and I still cannot promise that this will be the last time, so bear with me.

To latch, firstly, you need to get your baby to open his mouth very wide, and then he will reach out to cover your nipple and a large part of the areola. Next, your little one will use his tongue and lower jaw to form a tight seal over your nipple with his lips adequately turned out. Now to the part where he draws out milk successfully, the newborn uses his gum to compress the areola, and then he begins to move his tongue and jaw rhythmically in a sucking motion to draw out milk.

I am amazed every time we talk about the latching process. Why? It makes me wonder how a newborn does that much work to get milk from our breast. What do we expect to happen when our baby brings a feeding technique that does not require much hard work for her to feed?

Your baby does not necessarily have to master the proper way of latching on the nipple with a feeding bottle. What is even better is that it does not require any coordinated form of front-to-back tongue and jaw movement to stimulate your letdown reflex and to draw out milk. The most they need to do is suck the artificial nipple with their lips and gums, and then boom! The milk is out! Gravity can do quite a good job of getting the milk to drip without the baby touching the rubber nipple. Everybody, including your baby, loves being in control, and that is something your little one can easily enjoy from a bottle nipple. It gives them the power to control milk flow. If the milk is flowing too fast, all your baby has to do is thrust their tongue upward and forward to stop it!

Let us be honest; with all of these benefits we listed above, it is pretty logical that your baby would find it very hard to get back to latching on and sucking correctly from the breast after being given a chance to experience the wonders of feeding bottles. Now here is how the two concepts of nipple confusion and breast refusal play out with your baby.

Of course, we are pretty aware that artificial rubber or silicone nipples are of different sizes and textures from your breast nipples. Well, even your newborn acknowledges that fact. How? She tends to understand pretty fast that she does not have to struggle quite as hard to get milk from a bottle with an artificial nipple as she would from your breast. So, what happens? Instead, she would go for the bottle since It is a faster and more accessible means for her to get a full belly! We really cannot blame her, though!

Anyways, when you attempt to breastfeed your baby in this circumstance, she might protest the sudden change in the nipple texture size and even the ease in milk flow. We can say that she has gotten a different idea about what a nipple should feel like; she refuses your offer of being breastfed.

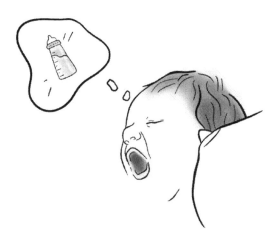

So, is this condition common with all babies?

84

I am glad you asked! Well, most babies might not have any problem switching from breast to a feeding bottle and back again. However, some babies, especially those who have not perfected the art of suckling at the breast, often find it hard to be efficient feeders, switching between the breast and the bottle and then back again. My midwife tried to help me avoid this effect during my first breastfeeding experience by advising that I should wait for about three weeks before initiating my baby into the whole bottle-feeding thing. Unfortunately, some of us do not have a choice but to do otherwise. However, there are ways we can navigate through it. We will discuss that in a bit.

Nevertheless, you must also understand that just as a baby can prefer artificial nipples to your breast nipples, some babies can exhibit the opposite reaction. How is that possible? They get so used to their mama's nipples that getting them to switch to the feeding bottle is almost impossible. But indeed, there are ways you can help your child adapt to create a balance because you deserve a break-even as a super mama!

HOW CAN I KNOW THAT MY BABY IS EXPERIENCING NIPPLE CONFUSION?

In most cases, when babies are experiencing nipple confusion, you would notice that they try to breastfeed with the same technique that they used when feeding on a bottle. Here are some of the signs you may have noticed in your baby's behavior.

- They become fussy at your breasts since the milk is not as instantly available as their feeding bottle.

- It becomes a big deal for them to do the usual one to

two minutes of breast sucking required to stimulate the letdown reflex.

- You may also observe that your baby refuses to open its mouth wide enough to get a proper latch. We know where that action came from, right? If you do use a feeding bottle, your baby does not necessarily have to open his mouth wide.

- Amidst grunting and arching, you might be successful in getting your baby to start sucking. However, he is likely to thrust his tongue up, which can push the nipple out of his mouth.

HOW DO I PREVENT NIPPLE CONFUSION AND BREAST REFUSAL?

I had several exciting but very enlightening conversations with different doctors and lactation consultants for this particular section. The first thing these experts made me realize was that nipple confusion and breast refusal were cases that demonstrated that prevention is better than cure. What does that even mean? The statement implies that it is easier for us as mamas to prevent our babies from getting into a confusing state or preferring their feeding bottles to our nipples. Fixing it after damage can be very difficult. Essentially, they said it was difficult and not impossible! But first, let us go through the steps you can take to prevent this from frustrating you.

All things being equal, the best way to prevent nipple confusion is to wait until your baby gets the hang of the latching and breastfeeding skills. Usually, it always takes about 3 to 6 weeks for your milk supply to be well-established and for your baby to have gained a good and safe amount of weight. When all of these are in place, you can comfortably break out the feeding bottle with little or no worries.

How then do you avoid nipple confusion and breast refusal when your doctor medically recommends that you give your baby supplement like instant formula quite early after their birth? For our first-time mamas, you should understand that getting those recommendations from your doctor may be because of your baby not gaining weight or breastfeeding a premature baby. It could also be because your baby has sucking issues like a tongue-tie. Other conditions can lead to this.

However, many mamas like us who find ourselves in this situation do not realize that we can be given these supplements in other ways that do not involve artificial nipples? Most of us tend only to bottle feed because it is the most common and convenient way. While this is true, bottle feeding is the method most likely to undermine your breastfeeding because it increases your baby's risk of developing nipple confusion or refusing to be breastfed once a bottle comes into the picture. Here are some alternative feeding options that do not involve artificial nipples. Notwithstanding, they are very effective methods to consider when feeding your baby with supplements or even expressed breast milk.

- **Finger feeding:** We might have mentioned this manual method of nursing as suitable solutions for situations when you have highly sore nipples or if you are having trouble getting your baby to latch on your breast. Well, news flash; finger feeding also works well when giving your baby supplements. Now how do you make it work? So basically, you will start by attaching the tube of the supplementing device to the tip of your finger. Afterward, you place that finger in your baby's mouth. So as your child sucks on your finger, the content of the instant formulas or whatever it might be will be drawn from the supplementing device into your child's mouth. You might not get it the first time you try it out. But with more practice and determination, you will get better at it!

- **Use a nursing supplementing device:** Have you ever heard of a device that helps you deliver supplements to your baby while she is latched onto your breast. It enables your baby to feed well while still stimulating your letdown reflex to increase your breast milk supply. So how exactly does this nursing supplementing device look? It comes in the form of a container that you can fill with your expressed milk or instant formula, and then the container has a tube attached to it that acts as a straw. So here is how it works. You secure the tube which is connected to the milk-filled container, to the tip of your nipple. So, as you breastfeed your baby, she draws out both milk from your breast with the additional content in the container. It is like killing two birds with one stone. I think this method is a great way to offer sufficient and additional nutritional support to your newborn with no chances of the supplement feeding interfering with your breastfeeding.
- If your baby is a little over 3 to 6 months, you can try feeding him with supplements using a sippy cup or a spoon.

WHAT TO DO WHEN MY BABY REFUSES TO BREASTFEED AFTER BEING INTRODUCED TO HER FEEDING BOTTLE?

When you find out that your baby is already showing signs of nipple confusion and breast refusal, you do not have to panic. Trust me; I know how frustrating and depressing it can be, especially if you want to breastfeed your baby exclusively. I was able to correct things for my last two children, so I know you can too! Here are a few tips that could be beneficial.

- If you can, ensure that you do not give up on breastfeeding. Stick to it! Or you could try to limit bottle sessions to when you are not around.
- Since you are already aware of all the hunger cues that your newborn is likely to exhibit, do not wait until things get to the point where your baby is ravenous to breastfeed. Delays will only make things worse.
- We said earlier that your baby could get frustrated because your milk is not as readily available as that of the bottle. Well, we can remedy that! Before you even try to get your baby to latch on and suck, you can stimulate your letdown reflex earlier by pumping a bit.
- To ensure you and your baby get back to being comfortable, you should practice the best breastfeeding techniques, be it your breastfeeding position or the way you get your baby to latch.
- Patience is a virtue that you must imbibe throughout these nursing sessions to make things right. Of course, I know both your emotions and that of your baby are high. You have every reason to be aggressive.

However, it would help if you were calm. Your baby will do the same if you manage to do this. So, take your time!

WHAT TO DO IF MY BABY REFUSES THE BOTTLE?

Surprisingly, nipple confusion and breast refusal can also happen the other way around where we find some mamas asking, "So Kim, I need a break from breastfeeding sometimes, but my baby just does not want to feed on the bottle?" Luckily for you, I have some tips that can be magic!

- **Get somebody close to stand-in:** Even though We have said earlier that breastfeeding is hard work for your little one, sometimes newborns can get attached to their mamas' nipples. So bad that even the idea of enjoying a more accessible and quicker option like a feeding bottle does not sit well with them. Sounds weird, right? Well, you might see things that way, but it seems so wrong to your baby. So when you as a mama offers milk in a bottle to your baby, what he might be thinking is, "How can I feed on this bottle when mama's breasts filled with juicy milk are right in front of me, even though she is hiding them from me all buttoned up!" Now That is the thought we need to erase from your baby's mind. So, let us try a different option.

Get someone else to offer your baby the feeding bottle. By doing this, it would be less tempting for your baby to reject the bottle. Who is in the best position to do a perfect job, though? Well, daddy could do the honors or your baby's grandma, Godmother, or even your close pal. Now I know some mamas might be scared that they will always need a mommy stand-in during their babies' feeding sessions with this option. Well, I am pleased to tell you that it is safe because the moment your little one gets the hang of her bottle, she would only care about filling her belly and not about the person giving it to her!

- **Experiment with different nipple types:** If your baby does not want to feed on a bottle, it could be that the nipple type, shape, or size is the problem. If one nipple type does not seem to be doing the job, go for another one. Take, for example, if you are using a rubber nipple, switch to silicone. The same thing applies to the size and shape of the artificial nipple. Essentially, ensure that you keep an eye on how fast the milk flows out. You do not want your baby to get frustrated, so the milk flow should be fast enough. However, it should not be so fast that your baby ends up choking. That would be a disaster! At least if you get one drop per second when you turn the bottle upside-down, that is okay.
- Increase bottle feedings as much as you can but while making a balance with breastfeeding. With every feeding session, take your time to observe your baby. Wait for what? Yes! By monitoring, you get to know what your baby wants. Some newborns often enjoy bottle feeding if you make it feel just like breastfeeding. But for others, they take to it quickly when you make the experience completely different. If the former is the case for your baby, you do not need to worry. However, if the latter is the case with your baby, then you can try switching your arms at different points during bottle feeding so that your baby has something different to feed her eyes. You can also do bottle feeding in other locations or different positions.

How do I balance bottle-feeding and breastfeeding?

Honestly, things would be so much easier if we, mamas, could stick to one of these two options. A simple all-or-nothing decision, right? Well, that is not possible. The reason is that even though we sometimes desire a break from breastfeeding or we find ourselves in situations where we cannot breastfeed, we all want to breastfeed our newborns exclusively to give them all the nutrients they need to grow healthy. Hence, we should work towards getting our babies to become efficient feeders in both areas. We can adopt techniques to create a balance between these two choices to enjoy the flexibility of both. You can focus on scheduling your baby's feeding sessions with a perfect mix of the two methods as well as the use of effective intervals. Getting an instant formula that your baby enjoys just as much as your breast milk can also make things very easy for both of you! Lastly, whether you are feeding your baby from your breast or a bottle, make sure that a lot of intimate skin-on-skin bonding characterizes your nursing time. So, interact with your little one!

No doubt, from what we have learned in this chapter, we can conclude that breastfeeding is hard work, not just for you as the mama but also for your baby. When your baby gets more comfortable with the idea of feeding on the bottle rather than your breast, it can be so frustrating. But trust me, your baby's refusal to be breastfed has nothing to do with you.

During those times, your emotions are high, and it is easy for you to make the wrong decision, but please do not! Seek the support of those you love and trust and block out all negativity. Keep reminding yourself that you are doing an excellent job of being a mama because that is what you are! As you do this, try to adopt the lessons we learned from this chapter as much as you can. Never forget that the goal is for your newborn to enjoy a splendid experience of breastfeeding without being forced to nurse!

PUMPING

I feel like this chapter is the most anticipated of all branches in this book, especially for our first-time mama. Well, first of all, I apologized for making you stay in suspense for a while. Okay, maybe I am not so sorry but trust me, I had the best intention in mind. I had to delay a little bit to sort out the basic yet most essential sections of breastfeeding.

Now, what is all this pent-up hype about pumping? I do not know if you can tell the excitement from my tone, but I am a fan of pumping milk; well, not as much as I am for exclusive breast-feeding. If you have followed my story so far, you will under-stand why I am grateful for breast pumps. Anyways, newbie mamas, I have a question for you. At least for once, have you ever heard a breastfeeding mama saying, "Oh! Thank God I pumped enough milk." I bet the Yes responses are more than the No! Well, sweethearts, the first thing you should know about pumping is that it is a lifesaving technique for every breast-feeding mama, and I am not exaggerating! My dear experienced mamas would agree that pumping is a versatile technique that you can use for so many reasons.

To start with, it is almost impossible for you as a mama to be with your baby, feeding her on demand 24 hours every day until your breastfeeding journey is complete and it is time to wean. Even if you do not have to go to work or head out at different times, you would eventually need a break from breastfeeding, and that is the point where a breast pump comes in to save the day. Please do not get me wrong; I recommend breastfeeding exclusively as much as possible. However, I would not pretend to be blind to situations that would arise when you cannot do the job as you wish you could. Hence, using a breast pump is an alternative but effective way you can take advantage to provide your baby with sufficient breast milk while still ensuring that you maintain a good milk supply.

For many mamas, especially our lovely first-timers, pumping often seems like an overwhelming and intimidating task, but it is not all that complicated. Ensure that you gain adequate knowledge about it. Then, you can go ahead to practice what you have learned as much as possible. Keep in mind that giving up is not an option for a super mama like you because once you know the proper techniques, you are good to go for life! Okay, maybe that is a little too much, but you get the point! So, take my hand as I walk you through answers to all the questions that are likely to come up in your thoughts when you hear about breast pumping.

WHY DO PEOPLE PUMP THEIR BREASTS FOR MILK?

I chose to start with this question about breast pumping because it was the first question that crossed my mind while I was breastfeeding my first born. As I said before, pumping is such a versatile technique that it works for so many reasons. Let us check some of those reasons that make mamas take up the offer of pumping.

- Let us start with me! I started pumping because I had

a low milk supply. In short, pumping helps me stimulate my letdown reflex more quickly so that my baby gets a good amount of breast milk. A breast pump can do wonders in helping you increase your milk supply.

- Sometimes, because of work or running errands, you might have no choice but to leave your newborn in the care of others, be it your family, friends, or a nanny. For this purpose, you can breast pump and store the milk so that your baby does not have to battle hunger while you are away.

- A mama with an overactive letdown reflex can also adopt breast pumping as a way of alleviating the pressure and reducing the amount of milk in her breast to ensure that her baby does not choke when he is breastfeeding. Then, she stores the rest for later.

- Mamas also pump when they find themselves in situations where their babies cannot latch or feed straight from their breast.

- Breast pumping can also be a valuable tool for mamas suffering from painful breast conditions like clogged ducts and mastitis. Remember that we mentioned that draining the breasts often can help speed up the healing process for these two conditions. Good! Breast pumps can work as an alternative or complementary tool with your baby's feeding to make things easier.

- Oh yes! Breast pumping can be your saving grace from leaking breasts and painful engorgement when your baby is not close to you!

- I know a few friends who pump for breast milk with the best and purest intentions. Can anybody guess? Well, they donate their milk to a milk bank or milk exchange program to feed babies who have lost their mothers or whose mamas cannot breastfeed them. Come on, how noble is that? Shout-outs to every mama doing the same! We are proud of you!

WHEN SHOULD I START PUMPING?

The best and only answer to this question is that you should start pumping when it is logical for you to start. I know what might be going through your mind right now, "what does that even mean?" Okay, let me make things clearer. The perfect time for you to start pumping depends highly on the kind of experience you are currently having in your breastfeeding journey. Every mother has a unique breastfeeding situation, so you should consider your situation exactly to know the right time. No stipulated time works for all mamas. "So, Kim, you are not going to be helping us here?" You know what? Let me try to give you a few illustrations, and then we will see if we all get it.

Some new moms start pumping very early, perhaps right there in the hospital or just a few days after getting home because of special reasons like them being unable to nurse because of your baby being premature or you having a deficient milk supply. Now That is the category where I belong!

For the other end of the spectrum, we already emphasized in the previous chapter that under normal circumstances, new moms should hold off on giving newborns bottles until they fully establish breastfeeding. We also know that pumping means you will have to feed your baby using a bottle unless you want to try the alternative feeding options, which do not involve artificial nipples. Anyways, due to this reason, other mamas often wait for about 4 to 6 weeks before they start pumping. At that time, breastfeeding would have been well-established, and you would be safe from your baby developing nipple confusion or breast refusal.

Another good thing is that, unlike the first few days, mamas are more likely to have enough time between feeding sessions to pump and store extra milk for their babies. I hope these illustrations clear things up for us too move on.

HOW DO I PUMP?

Enough of the preambles; this is the part we have all been waiting for, right? But first, I need to make sure you have the best and appropriate mindset for this learning process! Learning how to pump effectively can be pretty intimidating but let us discard the negative thoughts! You know why? These steps will ensure that you and your baby achieve success in the pumping game. Here we go!

START with ticking off all boxes on your hygienic checklist: At this point, we all know that it is ideal that we wash our hands before we breastfeed our babies, isn't it? The same thing applies to pumping. If you want to start on a safe note for every pumping session, you must ensure that you wash your hands thoroughly with soap and warm water. Many mamas do not know that the risk of their dirty hands infecting your baby is very high during pumping. Why? You do most of the job with your hands, so let us keep it clean.

Relax: Make sure that you get comfortable and relaxed both physically and mentally. There are so many diverse and fun ways you can do that. To begin with, you can get a quiet, comfortable place to sit. Solitude can do you lots of good. Doing yoga stretches or a simple meditation plan before every pumping session can also be of help. I know some of us might think that it is too much work. It can be entertaining, especially when it is your first experience at pumping. Beyond pumping, these activities can also benefit your mental health. How can I forget extra refreshment? Have a glass of water or a drink you like beside you, as the process can make you pretty thirsty!

FIND **a way to prepare your breast for a letdown:** Unlike what most mamas tend to assume, you do not just center your nipple in the flange opening and start to pump! The answer is negative. You do not necessarily have to stimulate your letdown reflex. However, it is advisable to get your breasts ready for a letdown before pumping. To do this, you can try massaging your breasts softly with your hands or a warm compress. Or you can also consider using some of the options we mentioned in a few chapters. When your baby is near, you can cuddle with her to launch the letdown. Still, if you are away from home, you can resort to looking at a picture of her or use your imagination to create a feeling of you holding her in your arms with her happy and cute nursing face beaming! This action might be crazy to anyone who has not experienced anything about motherhood but believes me, it does wonders.

ASSEMBLE **the pump kit and get centered:** Finding an effective pump is not a big deal, but what is more important is finding a flange that fits well, whether in shape or size. There is no room for compromising or improvising when it comes to the flange fit. If you are not using an electric pump, always make sure your pump has working batteries. As you center the flanges, you might want to focus on creating a good seal. Moistening the flange with water is a trick that works quite well for me. You can try it out too.

After you have gotten that preliminary task out of the way, you then place the flange over your breast and center the nipple in the flange opening! Every action should be done with caution. You might want to pump on both breasts at the same time to save time. All you have to do is to center the two flanges to each of your breasts; your fingers should be below the flanges, then your thumb will be placed on the top. As you adjust the dials on the breast pump, keep using one arm across both breasts to ensure an airtight seal. So that means that you would use your left hand to the right breast and the right hand to the left breast.

- **Turn on your pump and get to work:** Like how your baby nurses at the breast, most electric pumps usually begin the milk ejection process with a letdown phase. By starting with a shorter and quicker burst of suction, the pump somehow mimics the initial sucking that most babies do. Though it will take a few minutes for the letdown to happen afterward, the pump begins to operate normally.

Now let us talk about how to operate the dials! Always start pumping on a low suction but with high speed. After the letdown is complete and you see that your breast milk begins to flow, you can adjust the speed and suction to your comfort level. When you notice that the milk flow decreases but you are not done, you can adjust the speed to high until the subsequent letdown is over. Then you decrease the rate to medium when the milk flow increases, and like that, the cycle continues! Forget what anybody else said; pumping should not hurt at all! Once it begins to cause your pain, then you should stop because something is wrong.

- **Keep going:** Like any other technique that is of great essence, you will require a bit of practice, patience, focus, and determination to become an expert at breast pumping. You might not be able to express as much milk as possible at first, but with time, your body will learn to trigger your letdown reflex faster as you pump. With that, there will be an increase in the amount of milk you express during every pumping session.

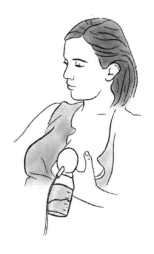

HOW LONG SHOULD I PUMP?

During the first few days into the pumping game, some mamas usually take up to 30 minutes with the pump to get a sufficient quantity of breast milk. However, on average, you should spend about 15 to 20 minutes pumping to collect a good amount of breast milk. If, after that, your breast does not feel well-drained to the point where the milk flow is not slowing down, then you can go ahead to spend a few more minutes. Just make sure you are not feeling pain.

HOW OFTEN SHOULD I PUMP?

When you are with your baby, you can schedule your pumping sessions between nursing sessions, usually every three to four hours. By doing that, you will be able to increase your milk supply while still aligning well with your baby's demand. On the other hand, you could be away from home and be trying to figure out how to pump as a way of making up for your baby's feedings that you missed! An excellent way to work around that is to pump using the same feeding schedule like the one you have back home.

HOW DO I STORE PUMPED MILK FROM MY BREAST?

The primary essence of breast pumping for most mamas is usually to store the milk for later. Thus, pumping for milk gets half of the job done! And you know what they say about a job being half-done; It is as good as no job done! Since we cannot afford to have our hard work go in vain, let us check out the effective and safe ways you can use to store breast milk.

To begin with, nowadays, many breast pumps usually come packaged in customized containers. You can use these containers both as feeding bottles or storage bottles for later. Some mamas often consider plastic bottles being too flimsy, so you can try collecting your pumped breast milk in those plastic bags that come with specific designs that are appropriate for storing breast milk. For this particular method, ensure that you only fill the bags only three-quarters full. That helps allow for expansion and prevents the milk from pouring out when you freeze them.

Reports show that breast milk can stay for around 4 hours when stored away from heat sources like the sun. That brings us to ask, 'What is a better option to preserve your milk from heat, other than storing it in the refrigerator *or* at room temperature?' Freezing is the best method to store your breast milk while still keeping it fresh. If you are using a freezer, you can even save your expressed milk for up to 6 months. I mean, how great is that? In all of this, make sure the milk is stored in small quantitics, at least 3 to 4 ounces. You can always keep as many containers as possible but ensure that you always start with the oldest milk when feeding your baby. How can you figure that out? Labeling them with the date on which you stored them can make the job easier for you.

HOW DO I KEEP MY BREAST PUMP IN CLEAN AND SOUND CONDITION?

We cannot overemphasize that maintaining hygiene is especially important during the early stage of your baby's birth, especially when using equipment like breast pumps. Suppose you leave your pump unclean with breast milk all over. In that case, there is a high possibility of getting contaminated germs into your milk, which can cause your newborn harm. As a result, you must always ensure that you disassemble all the pump parts immediately after using your breast pump and clean them thoroughly. Take your time with the process.

Start by scrubbing each part with a cleaning brush, liquid soap and hot water. Then you can end by rinsing them under running water. As you wash all these pump parts by hand, be sure that you do not place and wash them directly in the sink. A clean wash basin would be a safer and better option.

After washing and rinsing, you may then air-dry each part and put the pieces away when they are completely dried up. Sanitizing them daily or at least every two days should be your ideal goal. This option is specifically crucial for mamas whose babies have weakened immune systems or are just about three months old.

Also, take advantage of your dishwasher if your breast pumps are safe for use in that aspect. Place each of the disassembled parts in the top rack of your dishwasher, then set it on hot water and heat the drying cycle. And Viola! The job gets done!

. . .

EXTRA TIPS that can help you pumping and breastfeeding

We have already established that the perfect time to pump depends entirely on your breastfeeding situation. With time, you will figure out a pumping schedule that fits with that of your breastfeeding. Here are a few tips that can be of help.

- The best time to pump is when your breasts are ordinarily full. However, when you are missing feeding sessions because you are not close to your baby, it is best to pump at the exact times you usually nurse your baby, which is about 3 to 4 hours every day.
- Post-feeding pumping can also work for you. What this involves is for you to pump at the end of every nursing session. So, for example, if your baby sleeps off while being breastfed, you can use a manual pump to collect every last drop of the hindmilk.
- Your milk supply is likely to be very low late in the day due to exhaustion and stress. Thus, it is best if you do not pump during late afternoons or early evenings. Your mornings are your best bet to collect a sufficient amount of breast milk without getting tired out.
- Some weeks after I started pumping to feed my second child, I found out from my lactation consultant that some mamas can pump from one breast while their babies are breastfeeding on the other one. Eventually, I was also able to do this. It is a way of ensuring that you empty both breasts in a nursing session. So, on the one hand, your baby gets to fill his belly, and on the other hand, you can collect enough milk for storage later. Though this method is an efficient way to save time as a new mama, you

might want to pause a little before experimenting with this option. It is pretty tricky, and frustration is a state you cannot afford when pumping or breastfeeding.

And with that, we have made it to the end of breast-pumping 101! I bet the long wait was worth it. Pumping is never supposed to be painful, so do not try to endure it if it hurts. Stop the whole process and try again. This time, you should focus on getting every step right so that you can know the source or origin of the pain. Just as you have become an expert at latching and breastfeeding, I firmly believe that you would do a great job in pumping for the sake of your baby. It is not as daunting as it seems, so go for it and win, mamas! Your babies and I are cheering!

ALCOHOL, COFFEE, AND BREASTFEEDING

*T*he average time frame for pregnancy is nine months, but it could be a little longer for some mamas. Nevertheless, at a certain point, many of us, or perhaps even the whole mama squad, had to declare a partial or almost total break up with some of our favorite edibles and drinks. Alcohol and coffee fall into this category.

But first, I need to hear your views. Dear coffee and wine lovers in the house, how did you even manage to survive with just a minute or zero consumption of these things for nine entire months? I can hear some mamas already shaking their heads and saying, "Oh Kim! You do not want to know." Well, this proves again that we mamas deserve great accolades not just for hard work but also for our unwavering perseverance. Like superheroes, we fought hard and had a successful delivery. So, can anyone blame us if our first wish lists after birth have a cup of hot coffee or a glass of wine listed right at its very top!

Now, you finally get to go home from the hospital, and a few days or weeks later, you get the opportunity to fulfill your wish; perhaps, you went on a date with your partner or night hangout with your girls, and you want to relax with that glass of wine or cold beer served before you? But then, the big questions pop up in your head, "If it could affect me during my pregnancy, is this even safe for my breastfeeding baby? Should I drink or leave it? "

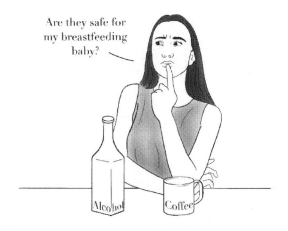

From another perspective, we cannot overemphasize the exhausting nature of breastfeeding, especially in the first few days of birth. During this stage, you have to wake up several times to feed your baby. Craving a cup of coffee to drive away sleep deprivation and swollen eyes is like a necessity. But again, the thoughts come up despite how tempting the aroma of the coffee bean is; it contains caffeine, so could it affect my baby? Such nobility and love for your little ones!

Anyways, due to these never-ending doubts and questions that mamas tend to have about drinking alcohol and coffee while breastfeeding, we will be wrapping this adventure up by uncovering the truth surrounding the consumption of these two controversial beverages. We will look at everything you need to know about drinking coffee and alcohol while nursing your newborn. Let us move!

IS IT SAFE FOR ME TO CONSUME COFFEE AND ALCOHOL WHILE BREASTFEEDING?

Shall we start with coffee since of the two beverages? It seems more subtle in effect? Unlike the negative assumptions that many mamas have about caffeine which is the dominant element in Coffee, the American Academy of Pediatrics has something different to say. According to this academy, caffeine is a maternal medication that works well with breastfeeding. The statement implies that drinking a moderate amount of coffee-containing caffeine can help increase your milk supply. That is good news!

Nonetheless, we must know that the information above does not guarantee safety if you consume excessive coffee. Of course, coffee is an effective tool to keep your eyes sharp at work or school after sleepless nights of breastfeeding. However, your consumption level of the beverages must fall within limits. Okay, so what are these limits? For each day, the standard recommendation is that you should consume less than 300 milligrams of caffeine. Now, do not look at me like that; the instruction was from medical experts who had carried out several studies to develop this safe amount for nursing mothers.

But how do you know if your coffee contains less than 300 milligrams of caffeine? Well, some experts have stipulated that you can get the total safe amount in two or three 8-ounces cups of coffee. Though this might be correct, this is not applicable for all coffee types. It is the type of coffee beans you are using and the time it takes to brew, which determines the exact amount of caffeine you will get in your coffee. But one thing is sure; for each cup of coffee, the caffeine content usually varies between 30 to 700 mg.

Notwithstanding all of the information we just mentioned, we have the verified information which states that lactating mothers do not have to break up again with coffee while nursing their babies. But please, if you can, do not forsake your sleep periods and try to make up for them by drinking coffee. Let us change gears!

Now about alcohol! If we were to consider this question to create 100% safety for our babies, then the perfect answer would be that complete abstinence from any alcoholic beverage is the best option for breastfeeding mothers. I can already feel the glares from many mamas, both seasoned and newbie, but you all need to calm down; I am just making an assumption. Now, let us get straight to the point.

So yes, it is safe to consume alcohol while you are on your breastfeeding journey. However, there are so many buts that come with this advantage. Your main guideline will be to practice the best kind of moderation! What does that even mean? It is simple. If you cannot help but take anything alcoholic, you will have to limit your intake to only one to two bottles in a week. The drinking spree has to be occasional.

These rules might sound a little too much, but we would all be grateful for them someday. Following these precautions, you get to ensure your alcohol consumption does not interfere with your neurological and coordination ability. Suppose the worst happens, and your sense of judgment suffers temporary impairment because of alcohol. In that case, there is a high tendency that you could make costly decisions and mistakes that may have a damaging effect on the growth, development, and even life of your newborn. And there is absolutely no way we would let that happen!

WHAT EFFECTS CAN MY CONSUMPTION OF ALCOHOL OR COFFEE HAVE ON MY BREASTFEEDING NEWBORN?

When you take these two drinks in moderate amounts, there is a very low possibility that your baby would be affected negatively. However, you should practice the only safe thing: after taking the coffee or alcohol, wait for about 2 or 3 hours before breastfeeding your babies. Why? A quick warning to answer this question. Well, we are about to launch into a long explanation that can be pretty confusing, so I was hoping you could stick with me with your full attention, and I promise you will get it.

Once you consume alcohol and coffee, the content moves freely with great speed from your bloodstream into your breast milk. Thus, there is no significant difference in the amount of alcohol and caffeine in your breast milk and bloodstream. Now the good news is that when you consume a moderate amount of either alcohol or coffee, most of the content would be entirely out of your body in about two to three hours. Now we know why the rule says you should breastfeed only about 2 to 3 hours after drinking coffee or alcohol, right?

Just a little bad news, though. This time range can vary depending on your body weight and composition, which is usually how fast your body will break down the substances. With this, we have confirmed again that occasional and moderate intake of coffee or alcohol is not something that can affect our babies.

Now, what happens when we don't follow the rules and go overboard with our alcohol or coffee intake? Things will undoubtedly go wrong, but we must remind ourselves that every baby is different and that some may be more sensitive to either alcohol or coffee. Another thing to consider in terms of effect is your baby's age.

Let us switch positions now and begin with the effects of drinking too much alcohol on your baby. So, mamas, have you ever heard someone say something like, "Oh dear! You are dealing with a low milk supply or letdown reflex. You know, you should try drinking one glass of wine or a bottle of beer in the evening at least twice a week." If you have, then I need you to ignore that advice completely. The most important thing to note here is that drinking alcohol has no beneficial effect on your milk supply and production. Instead, it can make things more difficult for them. Remember, we have discussed how the oxytocin hormone triggers the letdown reflex to make milk available for your little one. Recent research findings have proven that taking alcohol can hinder the release of the oxytocin hormones, which in turn inhibit your letdown and the release of milk to your baby. Quite an irony, isn't it? Alcohol offers the direct opposite of what most people claim it does.

Another effect of disobeying the rules concerning alcohol consumption is that its taste can reflect in your breast milk. Most babies do not like this. As such, it might lead to your baby refusing to breastfeed even when she is ravenous. If you are taking a lot of alcohol in the first few days or weeks of your baby's birth, then you are putting your newborn at a high risk of having liver damage. The increased risk is because, at that stage, her liver is immature, so that she would not digest the alcohol. This inability can breed a lot of adverse effects, including death. I am not trying to scare you but just stating facts.

Now, let us shift gears and look at the effects of coffee on breastfeeding. Consuming more than three to four cups of coffee in a day is already excessive. As such, it can have some side effects on your baby. If you have a premature baby or your newborn is just a few days or weeks old, the consequences could worsen. The result is because your premature baby or newborn absorbs and breaks down the caffeine content more slowly than you would expect if she was a little bit older. To let you know, that is not a good thing. Besides, it could be that your baby is more sensitive to caffeine than usual. Either way, the common side effects your baby might exhibit includes;

- She might not be able to sleep soundly and adequately as she should, especially at night. So you might notice that she keeps getting irritated and would wake up after shorter periods of sleep. Your petting techniques that used to have magical effects might no longer effectively get her to sleep.

- Due to her poor sleeping patterns, your baby might remain fussy all day long while constantly crying. As mamas, we tend to distinguish when our baby's cries are for food or something else. So, this should be easy for you to figure out.

- You also notice a difference in your baby's behavior in that she might be tense and jumpy for no reason.

WHAT AM I TO DO WHEN I HAVE DRUNK TOO MUCH ALCOHOL OR COFFEE?

From the devastating consequences we have learned so far, it is safe to conclude that excessive drinking of either coffee or alcohol is a prohibited area for every lactating mother. But somebody once told me "never say never." And I think what he meant was that because we are imperfect as humans, there would be times when we just cannot control whatever happens to us or those around us. You would agree that sometimes the best strategic plans often end up going the direct opposite.

To let you know, I am not trying to excuse any behavior. However, things often get out of hand when we want to unwind and take a break from the hard work of breastfeeding. This uncontrollable state is more familiar with alcohol than coffee. So, because we cannot take no chances, I have gathered a few tips that can help both you and your baby, even when you get so drunk to the point of vomiting or losing consciousness.

First of all, you must never breastfeed your baby in that drunken state. Being sober is a necessity. But how can you confirm if you are sober; Simple - if you can drive safely, you are sober. It could be that your breasts become full at that moment; express and drain the breast milk either with your hand or a pump. Doing this will help provide you relief and ensure that you do not tamper with your milk supply. However, you should not store the expressed milk from your intoxicated state to feed your baby with it. I know we have agreed that every drop of milk is gold but trust me, that particular one is only capable of causing damage.

Because I said we could express milk in our intoxicated state for relief, some experienced mamas might be wondering, "oh! So, you mean doing something like the pump and dump technique? NO! I am glad you raised this question. For our newbie mama, 'pump and dump' is a term used to describe a technique where you pump and drain your breasts of the milk claimed to have been impacted by alcohol or the caffeine content in your coffee. So basically, the assumption is that if you do this, you do not have to wait for 2 hours to feed your baby since you have gotten rid of the milk that has the alcohol or caffeine content. Well, news flash, mama, this technique of pumping and dumping milk does not in any way increase the rate at which the alcohol or caffeine moves out of your breast milk. It is only helpful in providing you with relief from engorgement pains and preserving your supple milk level.

The only valid technique you can adopt if you are concerned for your newborn is to enjoy your cup of coffee right after you nurse your baby. The logic behind this technique is that, pending your time before the next feeding session, there is a reduced chance of your baby consuming caffeine from your breast. That sounds like a more valid method, right.?

In the previous chapter, we talked about having a substitute mama for breastfeeding. Great! When you find yourself in an intoxicated state, ensure that you have someone else who will take care of your baby. It could be daddy, granny, or nanny. Most importantly, if you are drunk, you should not sleep on the same bed as your newborn. The same thing applies to any other sleeping location, including the couch or sofa. The reason for this is that when you are drunk, you have no control of your natural reflexes, so sharing a bed with your baby might not be a good idea.

At this point, we can call it a wrap on the alcohol, caffeine, and breastfeeding chapter! As you internalize all that we have learned in this final part of our adventure, I need you to keep in mind that no matter how new or experienced you are in the game of breastfeeding; you should take a break. Sometimes, after all the hard work and struggle that comes with being a mama, you deserve it! If you desire a cup of coffee, a glass of wine, or a cold bottle of your favorite alcoholic drink, feel free to indulge those desires once in a while. The paramount standard is for your every action and decision while relaxing to be moderate. I trust that you would do what is best for you and your little one!

AT THIS POINT, I would be incredibly thankful if you could just take 60 seconds to write a brief review on Amazon about how this book has helped you thus far, even if it's just a few sentences! I will love to read them all!

CONCLUSION

Wow! What an adventure! Writing this book has been one of the best decisions I have ever made in my life. I had such a great time through the comprehensive research, late nights, brainstorming, and refreshed memories. It was not so easy, but you know what helped? Every time I was getting tired, I would imagine that we were all sitting in a beautifully decorated room, having dinner as well as never-ending conversations and banter about motherhood. With that image in my heart, the words would flow freely! Even now, I have that image stored in the most sacred part of my heart, and I am sure that one day, we would get to make it a reality!

As an experienced mama of three, I have come to understand that our bodies are delicate and powerful pieces of machinery. They have the perfect design to notify, fix and correct most problems. However, most times, we mamas do not yield quickly enough to our bodies' signs to indicate a problem. Pain can be a good thing with lots of benefits. However, if there is one thing that I have repeatedly emphasized throughout every chapter of this book, then it would be that pain is neither normal nor something that we should ignore. It is our body's way of warning us that there is an issue.

Breastfeeding is an adventure that should be as comfortable as possible for both you and your baby. I understand that you might sometimes feel obliged to endure particular pain because you want to give your baby the best. But what if things eventually get out of control and you lose the ability to breastfeed your baby because your condition got worse. I sure hope none of us get to go through that kind of pain. Nevertheless, for that hope to become a reality, we must all learn to listen to our bodies. Paying attention to my body is a skill I have learned to master over time, and it has to help me ensure that I keep it in healthy and good shape.

I repeatedly emphasized that our mental health is just as important as our physical health during every breastfeeding stage. After a few mind-blowing sessions with my psychiatrist, I realized that all that matters was that my baby was growing healthy. Whether it is from formula or breast milk, it was not significant. The fact that I had to supplement could no longer affect how I felt! Do you know how I felt? Like the best mama in the world! Now I want you to understand something here – though my psychiatrist helped me through my depression, I had to change my mindset by my own will. If I had not summon the courage and transformed my perspective for the better at that point, I would not have even entertained the idea of writing a book to inspire and educate other breastfeeding moms.

In the introduction of this book, I made many promises, and I was determined to the end to fulfill all of them. I am glad that I was able to do just that. Now that you have learned and internalized the 9 bountiful secrets that can help you enjoy not only a pain-free breastfeeding experience but also ensure that your bond with your little one is on a more intimate and more profound level. It is left to you to incorporate every lesson you learned into your daily breastfeeding routine. You have the tools, and they are ready to be utilized. All that is left to do is for you to put them to good use; doing this will set you and your baby up for success throughout this journey.

Dear first-time mamas, it was a pleasure having you on this life-changing adventure. You are about to begin the journey of the most fantastic experience of your life. You have come so far, and I am proud of every one of you for your determination to learn and your desire to give your babies only the best! Even though I know the road will be anything but easy, I have complete assurance that you would conquer every challenge and emerge successfully.

My lovely seasoned mamas in the house, most of you picked up this book because you wanted to make the next breast-feeding experience better for yourselves and your babies. I am glad to say that you did it! Together, we learned new things while throwing our misconceptions and wrong assumptions into the trash. At different points when reading this book, we reminisced over our past experiences. I am smiling so hard right now because it was so worth it!

Whenever you find yourself wanting to give up, I sincerely hope that my story and the stories of other mamas would offer you the inspiration you need to remember just how brave and unique you are as a mother.

I know I have always expressed how super your mothering powers are, but I also want you to know that breastfeeding should not be a one-person job! As much as possible, you need to support the ones you love and trust! Many women have had similar experiences to yours and they can be of great help to your journey. So, how do you find this support system? You can simply join our Facebook and email community here.

When the going gets tough with no one to listen, understand or motivate you, this community of breastfeeding champions will always be there to give you strength with an extra dose of love and support. It is an emotional goodbye from me for now, but I will be waiting at the other side of the tunnel to celebrate with you when you win! Don't forget to join the community and share your progress with us!

GIVEAWAY

A FREE GIFT FOR OUR READERS!

Five adaptable recipes you can download and start your breastfeeding journey off on a delicious foot!! Visit this link

KimberlyNicoleWhittaker.com

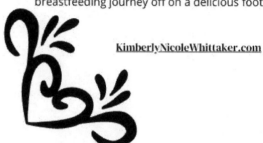

REFERENCES

References

Ameda (2020) Breast Pumping Guide: When and How Long to Pump. Retrieved from https://www.ameda.com/milk-101/milk-101-article/when-and-how-long-to-pump/

Austrian Breastfeeding Association. (2018). Let-down reflex (Milk Ejection Reflex). Retrieved from https://www.breastfeeding.asn.au/bf-info/early-days/let-down-reflex

Bonyata, K. (2018). Breastfeeding and Caffeine. Retrieved from https://kellymom.com/bf/can-i-breastfeed/lifestyle/caffeine/

Bonyata, K. (2018). How does milk production work? Retrieved from https://kellymom.com/hot-topics/milkproduction/

Bonyata, K. (2018). When will my milk come in? Retrieved from https://kellymom.com/ages/newborn/when-will-my-milk-come-in/

Bonyata, K. (2018). Breastfeeding Your Newborn — What To Expect In The Early Weeks. Retrieved from https://kellymom.com/hot-topics/newborn-nursing/

Bonyata, K. (2018). Latching and Positioning Resources. Retrieved from https://kellymom.com/ages/newborn/bf-basics/latch-resources/

Bonyata, K. (2018). Sore Nipples or Breasts? Here's Help. Retrieved from https://kellymom.com/hot-topics/sore-nipples-breasts/

Bonyata, K. (2018). Why are my nipples sore after months of pain-free nursing? Retrieved from https://kellymom.com/ages/older-infant/sorenipples-older/

Bonyata, K. (2018). Foremilk and Hindmilk – What Does This Mean? Retrieved from https://kellymom.com/bf/got-milk/basics/foremilk-hindmilk/

Bonyata, K. (2018). Breastfeeding and Alcohol. Retrieved from https://kellymom.com/bf/can-i-breastfeed/lifestyle/alcohol/

Britannica. (2019). Anatomic and Physiologic Changes In Other Organs And Tissue. Retrieved from https://www.britannica.com/science/pregnancy/Anatomic-and-physiologic-changes-in-other-organs-and-tissues

Carter, A. (2019). Fenugreek for Breast Milk: How This Magical Herb May Help with Supply. Retrieved from https://www.healthline.com/health/breastfeeding/fenugreek-breastfeeding

Cassoobhoy, A. (2020). Tongue-Tie. Retrieved from https://www.webmd.com/children/tongue-tie-babies

Cleveland Clinic. (2020). Breast Anatomy. Retrieved from https://my.clevelandclinic.org/health/articles/8330-breast-anatomy

DerSarkissian, C. (2019). Human Anatomy. Retrieved from https://www.webmd.com/women/picture-of-the-breasts

Dix, M. (2019). Is It Safe to Drink Alcohol While Breastfeeding? Retrieved from https://www.healthline.com/health/parenting/breastfeeding-and-alcohol

Greenfield, P and Fields L. (2011). 16 Things You Didn't

Know About Breastfeeding. Retrieved from https://www.parents.com/baby/breastfeeding/10-things-you-didnt-know-about-breastfeeding/

Higuera, V. (2018). Is My Let-down Reflex Normal? Retrieved from https://www.healthline.com/health/parenting/letdown-reflex#how-it-normally-works

Hohman, M. (2020). Breastfeeding Positions. Retrieved from https://www.whattoexpect.com/first-year/breastfeeding/positions/

Karen, M. (2018). Making Breast Milk: How Your Body Produces Nature's Perfect Baby Food. Retrieved from https://www.babycenter.com/baby/breastfeeding/making-breast-milk-how-your-body-produces-natures-perfect-ba_8785

Kanchan, S. (2020). Using Fennel While Breastfeeding – Does it Increase Milk Supply? Retrieved from https://parenting.firstcry.com/articles/using-fennel-while-breastfeeding-will-increase-milk-supply/?amp

Kainth, S. (2021). Deep Latch Technique – Benefits and How to Do. Retrieved from https://www.parenting.firstcry.com/articles/deep-latch-technique-benefits-and-how-to-do/%3famp

Kotlen, M. (2020). Breastfeeding and Nipple Confusion. Retrieved from https://www.verywellfamily.com/nipple-confusion-431932

Levine, H. (2020). Pumping Breast Milk Guide. Retrieved from https://www.whattoexpect.com/pumping-breast-milk.aspx

Levine, H. (2020). How to Treat Sore Nipples and Breastfeeding Pain. Retrieved from https://www.whattoexpect.com/first-year/breastfeeding/sore-cracked-painful-nipples-breastfeeding/

Madden, K. (2021). How to Get A Comfortable Deep Latch? Retrieved from https://balancedbreastfeeding.com/video-how-to-get-a-deep-latch/

Marcin, A. (2018). Is It Safe to Drink Coffee While Breast-feeding? Retrieved from https://www.healthline.com/health/parenting/coffee-and-breastfeeding

Mayo Clinic Staff, (2018). Tongue-Tie (Ankyloglossia). Retrieved from https://www.mayoclinic.org/diseases-conditions/tongue-tie/symptoms-causes/syc-20378452

Medela. (2020). When Does Breast Milk Come In? What to Look for and How You'll Know. Retrieved from https://www.medela.us/breastfeeding/articles/when-does-breast-milk-come-in-what-to-look-for-and-how-youll-know

Medela. (2020). 6 Breastfeeding Problems In The First Week – Solved. Retrieved from https://www.medela.com/breastfeeding/mums-journey/problems-newborn

Monica, S. (2018). Deep Latch Technique. Retrieved from https://www.pumpstation.com/blogs/articles/deep-latch-technique

Murphy, C. (2016). 5 Foods That Could Help Increase Your Breast Milk Supply. Retrieved from https://www.parents.com/baby/breastfeeding/tips/5-foods-that-could-help-increase-your-breastmilk-supply/

Murray, D. (2020). Breastfeeding Schedule for Your Newborn. Retrieved from https://www.verywellfamily.com/how-often-should-you-breastfeed-your-baby-431620

Murray, D. (2021). The Process of Making Breast Milk. Retrieved from https://www.verywellfamily.com/how-the-body-makes-breast-milk-4153170

Murray, D. (2021). How Garlic Affects Breastfeeding. Retrieved from https://www.verywellfamily.com/garlic-breastfeeding-and-increasing-breast-milk-supply-431840

Murray, D. (2020). Supplementing A Breastfed Baby. Retrieved from https://www.verywellfamily.com/alternative-feeding-methods-431905

Nonacs, R. Alcohol, And Breastfeeding: What are the risks?

Retrieved from https://www.contemporaryobgyn.net/view/alcohol-and-breastfeeding-what-are-risks

O'Connor, A. (2020). How to Get a Proper Breastfeeding Latch. Retrieved from https://www.whattoexpect.com/poor-breastfeeding-latch.aspx#

O'Connor, A. (2019). Nipple Confusion. Retrieved from https://www.whattoexpect.com/first-year/ask-heidi/nipple-confusion.aspx

Pearl Ben-Joseph, E. (2015). Breastfeeding FAQs: Pain and Discomfort. Retrieved from https://kidshealth.org/en/parents/breastfeed-discomfort.html

Pearson-Glaze, P. (2019). What is a Fast Letdown? Retrieved from https://breastfeeding.support/what-is-a-fast-let-down/

Pevzner, H. (2012). Can You Drink Alcohol While Breastfeeding? Retrieved from https://www.parents.com/baby/breastfeeding/basics/breastfeeding-and-alcohol/

Pitman, T. (2018). Ouch! How to Deal with Breastfeeding Pain. Retrieved from https://www.todaysparent.com/baby/breastfeeding/ouch-how-to-deal-with-painful-breastfeeding/amp/

Richardson, J. (2019). Breastfeeding FAQs: Getting Started. Retrieved from https://kidshealth.org/en/parents/breastfeed-starting.html

Sainani, S. (2020). Breastfeeding Pain – Causes and Solution. Retrieved from https://www.parenting.firstcry.com/articles/breastfeeding-pain-causes-and-solution/%3famp

Santos, M. (2018). Does Giving Your Baby a Bottle Cause Nipple Confusion? Retrieved from https://www.healthline.com/health/parenting/nipple-confusion

Sinrich, J. (2020). Caffeine While Breastfeeding. Retrieved from https://www.whattoexpect.com/first-year/breastfeeding/caffeine-while-breastfeeding/

Upstone, S. Butler, K. (2016). Positioning & Attachment.

Retrieved from https://www.laleche.org.uk/positioning-attachment/

US Center for Disease Control and Prevention. (2019). Breastfeeding and Alcohol. Retrieved from https://www.cdc.gov/breastfeeding/breastfeeding-special-circumstances/vaccinations-medications-drugs/alcohol.html

US Center for Disease Control and Prevention. (2019). How Much and How Often to Breastfeed. Retrieved from https://www.cdc.gov/nutrition/infantandtoddlernutrition/breastfeeding/how-much-and-how-often.html

Villines, Z. (2018). Can You Drink Coffee While Breastfeeding? Retrieved from https://www.medicalnewstoday.com/articles/322805

Wallis, M. (2020). Tongue-Tie: What It Is and How It is Treated. Retrieved from https://www.healthline.com/health/baby/tongue-tie#treatment

WIC Breastfeeding Support. (2020). How Breast Milk is Made. Retrieved from https://wicbreastfeeding.fns.usda.gov/how-breast-milk-made

WIC Breastfeeding Support. (2020). Steps and Signs of a Good Latch. Retrieved from https://wicbreastfeeding.fns.usda.gov/steps-and-signs-good-latch

ABOUT THE AUTHOR

I am a mother of 3: two stunning girls and a gorgeous boy.
I am writing this book because I realized that breast pain is one
of the main causes of mothers quitting breastfeeding. I have
always supported breastfeeding, even after I had a breast
reduction. Breastfeeding 3 children have taught me, and each
one has taught me something new. Right now, I want to share
every one of my experiences.
My passion is helping you become adequately prepared for
breastfeeding. It matters deeply to me because what you're
about to learn is what I wish I knew when I breastfed my first
baby.
As I continue to tandem breastfeed with my two youngest, I
realize how uneducated the vast public is on the topic. So, here
you go.
Hopefully, with this book, you will side-step all my mistakes!

Made in the USA
Columbia, SC
06 December 2021

50541285R00083